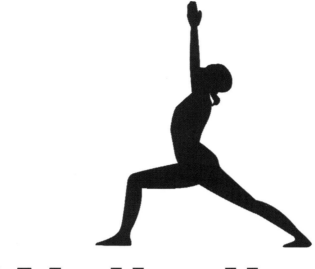

Wall pilates
workouts

for beginners

**30-Day Wall Pilates Challenge,
Only the most effective illustrated step-by-step exercises to
transform your body exercises for women and seniors**

Aurora Adams

Legal Notice:

This is a legal notice to inform you that the book titled WALL PILATES WORKOUTS FOR BEGINNERS authored by Aurora Adams is protected by copyright law. Any unauthorized distribution, reproduction, or use of the book, in whole or in part, is strictly prohibited and may result in legal action being taken against you. Under copyright law, the author has the exclusive right to reproduce, distribute, and publicly display the book. Any use of the book without the permission of the author or the publisher is a violation of their legal rights.

Disclaimer Notice:

The exercises and information contained within this book are intended for general guidance and should not be considered a substitute for professional medical advice, diagnosis, or treatment. It is crucial to consult with a healthcare provider or a qualified fitness instructor before commencing any exercise program, especially if you have underlying health concerns or medical conditions.

The author, Aurora Adams, and the publisher are not responsible for any injuries, health issues, or adverse consequences that may arise as a result of following the exercises, tips, or recommendations presented in this book. Every individual's physical condition and health requirements are unique, and it is essential to tailor any exercise program to your specific needs and limitations.

By using this book and engaging in the exercises described within, you acknowledge and accept full responsibility for your well-being and any associated risks. It is recommended to consult with a healthcare professional or fitness expert to ensure the exercises are safe and appropriate for your circumstances.

Aurora Adams

Table of Contents

Exercise Index

Introduction

Welcome to the world of Wall Pilates, a transformative approach to fitness that combines the principles of Pilates with the support of a wall. This book is your gateway to discovering a gentle and effective way to enhance your strength, flexibility, and overall well-being. Whether you're a complete beginner or someone looking to explore a new dimension of Pilates, you're in the right place.

Benefits of Wall Pilates for Beginners

Pilates is renowned for its focus on core strength, flexibility, and mindful movement. When combined with the support and resistance any simple wall can provide, these benefits are magnified, making Wall Pilates a fantastic choice for beginners. The wall becomes a steadfast partner, offering stability as you explore movements that help you connect with your body in a new way.

As a beginner, you might be apprehensive about trying a new fitness routine. Wall Pilates is here to welcome you with open arms. It's a low-impact, accessible practice that invites you to work at your own pace and gradually build confidence. The wall offers both guidance and challenge, making it easier to engage the right muscles and maintain proper alignment.

Safety Guidelines and Precautions

Before you embark on your Wall Pilates journey, it's important to understand a few safety guidelines and precautions. Always listen to your body and progress at a pace that feels comfortable. If you have any medical conditions or concerns, it's a good idea to consult with your healthcare provider before starting a new exercise program.

Throughout this book, we will guide you through a variety of exercises, each with clear instructions and modifications. It's essential to focus on proper form and alignment to ensure your safety and optimize your results. Remember that Rome wasn't built in a day, and your progress is what matters most.

Get ready to experience the joy of Wall Pilates, where the wall becomes your partner in achieving your fitness goals. We're excited to accompany you on this journey as you discover a new level of strength, flexibility, and mind-body connection. Let's dive in and begin your Wall Pilates adventure!

Wall Pilates Workouts for Beginners

Getting Started with Wall Pilates

Welcome to the beginning of your journey! This chapter is all about laying a solid foundation as you step into the world of Pilates and explore the unique benefits of practicing against a wall. Whether you're a complete novice or have some fitness experience, this chapter will provide the insights you need to start your current adventure on the right foot.

What is Pilates?

Pilates is a holistic approach to fitness that focuses on strengthening the core, improving flexibility, and enhancing overall body awareness. Developed by Joseph Pilates in the early 20th century, this method combines controlled movements, breath, and mindfulness to create a balanced and aligned body.

Understanding Wall Pilates

Wall Pilates takes the traditional principles of the practice and adds a new dimension by incorporating the support and resistance of a wall. This makes it an ideal starting point for beginners who may feel more comfortable with added stability. The wall acts as a constant reference point, guiding you in maintaining proper alignment and engaging the right muscles.

Benefits of Wall Pilates for Beginners

The benefits of Wall Pilates for beginners are abundant:

1. **Stability and Support**: The wall provides stability, making it easier for beginners to focus on form and technique without feeling overwhelmed.

2. **Gentle on Joints**: It is low-impact, reducing stress on joints and minimizing the risk of injury.

3. **Core Strength**: Core engagement is a fundamental aspect of Pilates in general, and the use of the wall encourages you to connect with your core muscles effectively.

4. **Flexibility**: The wall helps you achieve better alignment, which can lead to improved flexibility and reduced muscle tension.

5. **Mind-Body Connection**: It encourages mindful movement and body awareness, fostering a deeper connection between your body and mind.

Preparing for Your Wall Pilates Journey

Before you jump into your Wall Pilates workouts, it's important to set yourself up for success:

1. **Clear Space**: Choose a space with enough room for you to move comfortably and safely. Make sure the wall you're using is free of obstacles.

2. **Attire**: Wear comfortable, breathable clothing that allows you to move freely. Avoid anything too loose or restrictive.

3. **Equipment**: For most of these exercises, you won't need any special equipment. Just a clear wall space and perhaps a yoga mat for added comfort.

4. **Mindset**: Approach your practice with an open mind and a willingness to learn. Be patient with yourself and focus on the journey rather than achieving perfection.

As you dive into the subsequent chapters, you'll explore various Wall Pilates exercises designed specifically for beginners. Each exercise will be accompanied by clear instructions, modifications, and tips to ensure your safety and progress. Remember, this is a personal journey, and the more you put into it, the more you'll get out of it. So, let's get ready to experience its joy and benefits!

Basics of Wall Pilates Exercises

In this chapter, you'll delve into the fundamental aspects of our proposed exercises. You'll learn about the importance of proper breathing techniques, core engagement, and the unique role that the wall plays in supporting and enhancing your practice. These foundational elements will serve as the building blocks for your Wall Pilates journey, allowing you to progress confidently and safely.

Proper Breathing Techniques

Breathing is a cornerstone of the practice, and it's crucial to understand how to breathe effectively during your exercises. The goal is to cultivate mindful breathing that supports your movements and encourages relaxation. Here's a simple guideline for breathing in your workout:

- Inhale: through your nose, filling your lungs with air and expanding your ribcage.
- Exhale: through pursed lips, engaging your core muscles as you draw your navel towards your spine.

Remember that the breath should flow naturally, and you should avoid holding it during exercises. Coordinating your breath with your movements will help you maintain stability and focus.

Core Engagement and Alignment

Core engagement is a fundamental principle in Pilates, and it's essential for maintaining proper alignment and stability during the exercises. The core encompasses not only your abdominal muscles but also your back and pelvic floor muscles. Engaging your core provides a stable foundation for movement and helps protect your spine.

To engage your core:

- Imagine pulling your belly button towards your spine without holding your breath.
- Gently activate your pelvic floor muscles.
- Maintain this engagement throughout your exercises to support your posture and movements.

The Role of the Wall: Support and Resistance

One of the unique aspects of Wall Pilates is the support and resistance that the wall provides. The wall acts as a reference point, helping you maintain proper alignment and form. It offers stability, especially for beginners who might need additional support as they build their strength and flexibility.

Additionally, the wall can provide a gentle form of resistance. When you press into the wall or use it for leverage, you engage your muscles more effectively, making the exercises more challenging and effective.

Understanding how to use the wall as a tool for support and resistance will enhance your Wall Pilates experience and help you achieve better results.

As you progress through your journey, these basic principles of breathing, core engagement, and utilizing the wall's support and resistance will gradually become second nature. The following chapters will take you step by step through a variety of Wall Pilates exercises, each with its unique benefits and challenges. With these foundations in place, you're well-equipped to dive into the world of Wall Pilates with confidence and enthusiasm.

Wall Pilates Warm-Up

A proper warm-up is essential before engaging in any exercise routine, including Wall Pilates. Warming up prepares your body for movement, increases blood flow to your muscles, and reduces the risk of injury. In this chapter, you'll discover a series of gentle and effective warm-up exercises that are specifically designed to prepare you for your Wall Pilates practice.

Neck and Shoulder Rolls
1. Stand or sit comfortably, facing the wall.
2. Gently drop your chin to your chest and slowly roll your head in a circular motion to one side.
3. Continue the circular motion, bringing your ear towards your shoulder, then gently rolling your head back, and finally returning to the starting position.
4. Repeat the same motion in the opposite direction.

Arm Circles
1. Stand facing the wall with your feet hip-width apart.
2. Extend your arms out to the sides at shoulder height.
3. Start making small circles with your arms, gradually increasing the size of the circles.
4. After a few circles, reverse the direction in which you do them.

Standing Side Stretches
1. Stand with your right side facing the wall.
2. Raise your right arm overhead and lean towards the left, creating a gentle side stretch.
3. Feel the stretch along your right side from your hip to your fingertips.
4. Hold for a few breaths, then switch sides and repeat the stretch on the left.

Benefits of a Warm-Up:
- **Increased Blood Flow:** Warm-up exercises increase circulation, ensuring that your muscles receive more oxygen and nutrients, which enhances their performance.
- **Joint Lubrication:** Moving your joints through a full range of motion in the warm-up helps lubricate the joints and reduce stiffness.
- **Mental Preparation:** Warm-ups also mentally prepare you for your practice, allowing you to shift your focus from the outside world to your body and breath.

A proper warm-up doesn't have to be time-consuming, but it is crucial for ensuring a safe and effective workout. Spend a few minutes engaging in these warm-up exercises before moving on to the Wall Pilates ones in the subsequent chapters. By doing so, you'll set the stage for a productive and enjoyable session that supports your well-being and progress.

28-day basic program for beginners

Week 1: Building Core Awareness and Mobility

Day 1:

1. Wall Roll Down: 2 sets of 6 repetitions
2. Wall Pike: Hold for 10 seconds, rest for 10 seconds; repeat 3 times
3. Wall Bridge: 2 sets of 8 repetitions
4. Wall Arm Circles: 2 sets of 10 repetitions
5. Wall Split Stretch: 2 sets of 6 repetitions

Day 2:

1. Wall Squats: 3 sets of 10 repetitions
2. Wall Plank: Hold for 15 seconds, rest for 10 seconds; repeat 3 times
3. Wall Side Leg Lifts: 2 sets of 8 repetitions on each leg
4. Wall Lunge Stretch: Hold for 20 seconds on each leg; repeat 2 times
5. Wall Push-Ups: 2 sets of 8 repetitions

Day 3: Rest and Recovery
Day 4:

1. Wall Pike: Hold for 12 seconds, rest for 8 seconds; repeat 4 times
2. Wall Teaser: 2 sets of 6 repetitions
3. Wall Scissor: 2 sets of 10 repetitions on each leg
4. Wall Triceps Dips: 2 sets of 8 repetitions
5. Wall Split Stretch: 2 sets of 6 repetitions

Day 5:

1. Wall Single Leg Stretch: 2 sets of 8 repetitions on each leg
2. Wall Torso Rotation: 2 sets of 10 repetitions on each side
3. Wall Side Plank: Hold for 15 seconds on each side; repeat 2 times
4. Wall Split Stretch: Hold for 20 seconds on each leg; repeat 2 times
5. Wall Back Extension: 2 sets of 8 repetitions

Day 6: Rest and Recovery

Day 7:

1. Wall Pike: Hold for 15 seconds, rest for 10 seconds; repeat 4 times
2. Wall Arabesque: 2 sets of 10 repetitions on each leg
3. Wall Push-Up with Leg Lift: 2 sets of 8 repetitions
4. Wall Calf Stretch: Hold for 30 seconds on each leg; repeat 2 times
5. Wall Mermaid Stretch: Hold for 20 seconds on each side; repeat 2 times

Week 2: Developing Strength and Balance

Day 8-14:

Repeat the exercises from Week 1 with an increase in repetitions or hold times where indicated. Aim to perform 3 sets of each exercise and gradually challenge yourself to deepen your engagement and control.

Week 3: Increasing Intensity and Coordination

Day 15-21:

Continue repeating the exercises from Weeks 1 and 2, focusing on performing 3 sets with increased repetitions or longer hold times. Add 1-2 repetitions or 5-second increments to the hold times to progressively challenge yourself.

Week 4: Mastery and Progression

Day 22-28:

Continue with the exercises from previous weeks, increasing the intensity by adding an extra set to each exercise. You can also experiment with combining exercises for a more dynamic flow.

Day 29-30:

Repeat the entire program from Week 4, focusing on quality over quantity. Pay attention to your form and mindfulness in each movement.

Congratulations on completing your 4-week beginner's program! This program is designed to gradually introduce you to the world of Wall Pilates, helping you build a strong core, enhance your flexibility, and improve your overall body awareness. As you progress, you can continue practicing these exercises and gradually increase the intensity to challenge yourself further. Remember to listen to your body, stay consistent, and enjoy the journey of self-discovery and growth through Wall Pilates.

28-day Posture Support Program

Welcome to the 4-week Posture Support Program! This program is tailored to help you enhance your posture while strengthening your core and promoting overall body alignment. By incorporating a variety of Wall Pilates exercises, you'll work towards achieving better posture and increased body awareness. Let's get started on your journey to improved posture!

Week 1: Core Awareness and Mobility

Day 1:

1. Wall Roll Down: 2 sets of 6 repetitions
2. Wall Squats: 3 sets of 10 repetitions
3. Wall Angel: 2 sets of 10 repetitions
4. Wall Bridge: 2 sets of 8 repetitions
5. Handstand against a wall: 1 set of 10-20 seconds

Day 2:

1. Wall Plank: Hold for 15 seconds, rest for 10 seconds; repeat 3 times
2. Wall Side Leg Lifts: 2 sets of 8 repetitions on each leg
3. Wall Single Leg Stretch: 2 sets of 6 repetitions on each leg
4. Wall Corkscrew: 2 sets of 8 repetitions
5. Handstand against a wall: 1 set of 10-20 seconds

Day 3: Rest and Recovery

Day 4:

1. Wall Pike: Hold for 12 seconds, rest for 8 seconds; repeat 4 times
2. Wall Push-Ups: 2 sets of 8 repetitions
3. Wall Pike Roll Down: 2 sets of 6 repetitions
4. Wall Reverse Plank: Hold for 15 seconds, rest for 10 seconds; repeat 3 times
5. Handstand against a wall: 1 set of 10-20 seconds

Day 5:

1. Wall Scissor: 2 sets of 10 repetitions on each leg
2. Wall Arm Circles: 2 sets of 10 repetitions
3. Wall Side Plank: Hold for 15 seconds on each side; repeat 2 times
4. Wall Lunge Stretch: Hold for 20 seconds each leg; repeat 2 times
5. Handstand against a wall: 1 set of 10-20 seconds

Day 6: Rest and Recovery

Day 7:

1. Wall Arabesque: 2 sets of 10 repetitions on each leg

2. Wall Torso Rotation: 2 sets of 10 repetitions on each side

3. Wall Back Extension: 2 sets of 8 repetitions

4. Wall Chest Opener: Hold for 20 seconds; repeat 2 times

5. Handstand against a wall: 1 set of 10-20 seconds

Week 2: Strengthening and Balancing

Day 8-14:

Repeat the exercises from Week 1 with an increase in repetitions or hold times where indicated. Aim to perform 3 sets of each exercise and gradually challenge yourself to deepen your engagement and control.

Week 3: Advancing Postural Control

Day 15-21:

Continue repeating the exercises from Weeks 1 and 2, focusing on performing 3 sets with increased repetitions or longer hold times. Add 1-2 repetitions or 5-second increments to the hold times to progressively challenge yourself.

Week 4: Mastering Postural Alignment

Day 22-28:

Continue with the exercises from previous weeks, increasing the intensity by adding an extra set to each exercise. You can also experiment with combining exercises for a more dynamic flow.

Day 29-30:

Repeat the entire program from Week 4, focusing on quality over quantity. Pay attention to your posture, your alignment, and in using mindfulness in each movement.

Congratulations on completing the 4-week Posture Support Program! By dedicating yourself to this program, you're taking significant steps towards achieving better posture, enhanced core strength, and overall body awareness. As you progress, continue practicing these exercises to maintain and further improve your posture. Remember that consistent effort and mindful practice are key to long-lasting benefits.

28-day Body Shaping and Butt Firming Program

Welcome to the 4-week Body Shaping and Butt Firming Program! This program is designed to help you sculpt your body, firm your butt, and increase overall muscle tone using a combination of targeted Wall Pilates exercises. By focusing on specific movements, you'll work towards achieving a more toned and defined physique. Let's begin your journey to a firmer and more shapely body!

Week 1: Building Core Strength and Butt Activation

Day 1:

1. Wall Roll Down: 2 sets of 6 repetitions
2. Wall Squats: 3 sets of 10 repetitions
3. Wall Bridge: 2 sets of 8 repetitions
4. Wall Pike: Hold for 10 seconds, rest for 10 seconds; repeat 3 times
5. Handstand against a wall: 1 set of 10-20 seconds

Day 2:

1. Wall Single Leg Stretch: 2 sets of 8 repetitions on each leg
2. Wall Side Leg Lifts: 2 sets of 10 repetitions on each leg
3. Wall Scissor: 2 sets of 10 repetitions on each leg
4. Wall Push-Ups: 2 sets of 8 repetitions
5. Handstand against a wall: 1 set of 10-20 seconds

Day 3: Rest and Recovery
Day 4:

1. Wall Split Stretch: 2 sets of 6 repetitions
2. Wall Hip Abduction: 2 sets of 12 repetitions on each leg
3. Wall Lunge Stretch: Hold for 20 seconds on each leg; repeat 2 times
4. Wall Push-Up with Leg Lift: 2 sets of 8 repetitions
5. Wall Squats: 3 sets of 8 repetitions
6. Handstand against a wall: 1 set of 10-20 seconds

Day 5:

1. Wall Teaser: 2 sets of 6 repetitions
2. Wall Corkscrew: 2 sets of 8 repetitions
3. Wall Arm Circles: 2 sets of 10 repetitions

4. Wall Reverse Plank: Hold for 15 seconds, rest for 10 seconds; repeat 3 times

5. Handstand against a wall: 1 set of 10-20 seconds

Day 6: Rest and Recovery

Day 7:

1. Wall Arabesque: 2 sets of 10 repetitions on each leg

2. Wall Side Plank: Hold for 15 seconds on each side,; repeat 2 times

3. Wall Triceps Dips: 2 sets of 8 repetitions

4. Wall Split Squat: 2 sets of 10 repetitions on each leg

5. Handstand against a wall: 1 set of 10-20 seconds

Week 2: Progressive Butt Firming and Core Activation

Day 8-14:

Repeat the exercises from Week 1 with an increase in repetitions or hold times where indicated. Aim to perform 3 sets of each exercise and gradually challenge yourself to deepen your engagement and control.

Week 3: Advanced Shaping and Muscle Toning

Day 15-21:

Continue repeating the exercises from Weeks 1 and 2, focusing on performing 3 sets with increased repetitions or longer hold times. Add 1-2 repetitions or 5-second increments to the hold times to progressively challenge yourself.

Week 4: Sculpting and Shaping Mastery

Day 22-28:

Continue with the exercises from previous weeks, increasing the intensity by adding an extra set to each exercise. You can also experiment with combining exercises for a more dynamic flow.

Day 29-30:

Repeat the entire program from Week 4, focusing on quality over quantity. Pay attention to your form, engagement, and mindfulness in each movement.

Congratulations on completing the 4-week Body Shaping and Butt Firming Program! By dedicating yourself to this program, you're taking significant steps towards achieving a more sculpted and toned body. As you progress, continue practicing these exercises to maintain and further improve your muscle tone and body shape. Remember that consistent effort, proper nutrition, and mindful practice are key to achieving your desired results.

28-day Maximum Effective Weight Loss Program

Welcome to the 4-week Maximum Effective Weight Loss Program! This program is designed to help you accelerate your weight loss journey by combining high-intensity cardio exercises with targeted strength training. The selected Wall Pilates exercises will engage multiple muscle groups while keeping your heart rate up for optimal fat burning. Get ready to shed those pounds and achieve your weight loss goals!

Week 1: Building Stamina and Core Activation

Day 1:

1. Wall Roll Down: 2 sets of 6 repetitions
2. Wall Squats: 3 sets of 12 repetitions
3. Wall Plank: Hold for 15 seconds, rest for 10 seconds; repeat 3 times
4. Wall Scissor: 2 sets of 12 repetitions on each leg
5. Handstand against a wall: sets of 10-20 seconds

Day 2:

1. Wall Pike: Hold for 12 seconds, rest for 8 seconds; repeat 4 times
2. Wall Push-Ups: 3 sets of 10 repetitions
3. Wall Side Leg Lifts: 2 sets of 12 repetitions on each leg
4. Wall Arm Circles: 2 sets of 12 repetitions
5. Handstand against a wallet set of 10-20 seconds

Day 3: Rest and Recovery
Day 4:

1. Wall Bridge: 2 sets of 10 repetitions
2. Wall Split Stretch: 2 sets of 6 repetitions
3. Wall Hip Abduction: 2 sets of 15 repetitions on each leg
4. Wall Push-Up with Leg Lift: 2 sets of 10 repetitions
5. Handstand against a wall: 1 set of 10-20 seconds

Day 5:

1. Wall Reverse Plank: Hold for 15 seconds, rest for 10 seconds; repeat 3 times
2. Wall Single Leg Stretch: 2 sets of 10 repetitions on each leg
3. Wall Teaser: 2 sets of 6 repetitions

4. Wall Side Plank: Hold for 20 seconds on each side; repeat 2 times

5. Handstand against a wall: 1 set of 10-20 seconds

Day 6: Rest and Recovery

Day 7:

1. Wall Split Squat: 2 sets of 12 repetitions on each leg

2. Wall Corkscrew: 2 sets of 10 repetitions

3. Wall Triceps Dips: 2 sets of 12 repetitions

4. Wall Split Stretch: Hold for 25 seconds on each leg; repeat 2 times

5. Handstand against a wall: 1 set of 10-20 seconds

Week 2: Intensifying Cardio and Muscle Engagement

Day 8-14:

Repeat the exercises from Week 1 with an increase in repetitions or hold times where indicated. Aim to perform 3 sets of each exercise and gradually challenge yourself to deepen your engagement and control.

Week 3: Boosting Fat Burning and Strength

Day 15-21:

Continue repeating the exercises from Weeks 1 and 2, focusing on performing 3 sets with increased repetitions or longer hold times. Add 1-2 repetitions or 5-second increments to the hold times to progressively challenge yourself.

Week 4: Igniting Weight Loss and Full-Body Toning

Day 22-28:

Continue with the exercises from previous weeks, increasing the intensity by adding an extra set to each exercise. You can also experiment with combining exercises for a more dynamic flow.

Day 29-30:

Repeat the entire program from Week 4, focusing on quality over quantity. Push your limits while maintaining proper form and mindful movement.

Congratulations on completing the 4-week Maximum Effective Weight Loss Program! By committing to this program, you're taking significant steps towards achieving your weight loss goals. Remember to pair your workouts with a balanced diet and stay hydrated. Consistency, determination, and mindful exercise are key to maximizing your weight loss results. Enjoy your journey to a healthier and fitter you!

28-day Easy Mood Improvement and Stress Relief Program

Welcome to the 4-week Easy Mood Improvement and Stress Relief Program! This program is designed to help you experience calmness and uplift your mood through gentle and accessible Wall Pilates exercises. By focusing on easy-to-follow movements and relaxation techniques, you'll find relief from stress and promote emotional well-being. Let's start your journey to a more peaceful and joyful you!

Week 1: Gentle Movement and Relaxation

Day 1:

1. Wall Roll Down: 2 sets of 6 repetitions
2. Wall Squats: 2 sets of 8 repetitions
3. Wall Bridge: 2 sets of 6 repetitions
4. Wall Arm Circles: 2 sets of 8 repetitions
5. Handstand against a wall: 1 set of 10-20 seconds

Day 2:

1. Wall Plank: Hold for 10 seconds, rest for 10 seconds; repeat 3 times
2. Wall Side Leg Lifts: 2 sets of 6 repetitions on each leg
3. Wall Lunge Stretch: Hold for 15 seconds each leg; repeat 2 times
4. Wall Chest Opener: Hold for 15 seconds; repeat 2 times

Day 3: Rest and Reflection
Day 4:

1. Wall Split Stretch: 2 sets of 6 repetitions
2. Wall Hip Abduction: 2 sets of 10 repetitions on each leg
3. Wall Triceps Dips: 2 sets of 6 repetitions
4. Wall Oblique Twist: 2 sets of 8 repetitions on each side
5. Handstand against a wall: 1 set of 10-20 seconds

Day 5:

1. Wall Pike: Hold for 8 seconds, rest for 8 seconds; repeat 4 times
2. Wall Single Leg Stretch: 2 sets of 6 repetitions on each leg

3. Wall Mermaid Stretch: Hold for 15 seconds each side; repeat 2 times

4. Wall Back Extension: 2 sets of 6 repetitions

Day 6: Rest and Rejuvenation

Day 7:

1. Wall Arabesque: 2 sets of 8 repetitions on each leg

2. Wall Teaser: 2 sets of 4 repetitions

3. Wall Corkscrew: 2 sets of 6 repetitions

4. Wall Split Stretch: Hold for 20 seconds on each leg; repeat 2 times

5. Handstand against a wall: 1 set of 10-20 seconds

Week 2: Serenity and Mindful Movement

Day 8-14:

Repeat the exercises from Week 1 with an increase in repetitions or hold times where indicated. Focus on breathing deeply and mindfully throughout your practice.

Week 3: Inner Peace and Gentle Strengthening

Day 15-21:

Continue repeating the exercises from Weeks 1 and 2, aiming for a soothing practice. Prioritize relaxation and gentle engagement.

Week 4: Tranquility and Emotional Balance

Day 22-28:

Continue with the exercises from previous weeks, adjusting the intensity to your comfort level. Embrace each movement as an opportunity for self-care and stress relief.

Day 29-30:

Repeat the entire program from Week 4, emphasizing self-kindness and gratitude. Focus on how each movement contributes to your emotional well-being.

Congratulations on completing the 4-week Easy Mood Improvement and Stress Relief Program! By dedicating yourself to this program, you're nurturing your mental and emotional wellness. Remember that it's okay to modify exercises to match your comfort level. Allow these simple exercises to be a sanctuary of peace and positivity in your daily life.

28-day Easy Senior Fitness Program

This program is designed to promote flexibility, balance, and overall fitness for seniors through a series of gentle Wall Pilates exercises. Please consult with a healthcare professional before starting any exercise program, especially if you have existing health concerns.

Week 1: Gentle Introduction

Day 1:

1. Wall Roll Down: 2 sets of 4 repetitions
2. Wall Squats: 2 sets of 6 repetitions
3. Wall Arm Circles: 2 sets of 6 repetitions
4. Wall Chest Opener: Hold for 10 seconds; repeat 2 times
5. Handstand against a wall: 1 set of 10-20 seconds

Day 2:

1. Wall Bridge: 2 sets of 4 repetitions
2. Wall Lunge Stretch: Hold for 10 seconds each leg; repeat 2 times
3. Wall Single Leg Stretch: 2 sets of 4 repetitions on each leg
4. Wall Calf Stretch: Hold for 10 seconds; repeat 2 times

Day 3: Rest and Recovery
Day 4:

1. Wall Side Leg Lifts: 2 sets of 4 repetitions for each leg
2. Wall Split Stretch: Hold for 10 seconds each leg; repeat 2 times
3. Wall Plank: Hold for 10 seconds, rest for 10 seconds; repeat 2 times
4. Wall Back Extension: 2 sets of 4 repetitions
5. Handstand against a wall: 1 set of 10-20 seconds

Day 5:

1. Wall Pike: Hold for 6 seconds, rest for 6 seconds; repeat 3 times
2. Wall Hip Abduction: 2 sets of 6 repetitions on each leg
3. Wall Side Plank: Hold for 10 seconds on each side; repeat 2 times
4. Wall Arabesque: 2 sets of 4 repetitions on each leg

Day 6: Rest and Recovery

Day 7:

1. Wall Push-Ups: 2 sets of 6 repetitions

2. Wall Oblique Twist: 2 sets of 6 repetitions on each side

3. Wall Corkscrew: 2 sets of 4 repetitions

4. Wall Mermaid Stretch: Hold for 10 seconds each side; repeat 2 times

5. Handstand against a wall: 1 set of 10-20 seconds

Week 2: Increasing Mobility and Balance

Day 8-14:

Repeat the exercises from Week 1 with an increase in repetitions or hold times where indicated. Focus on stability, control, and gradual improvement.

Week 3: Building Strength and Flexibility

Day 15-21:

Continue with the exercises from Weeks 1 and 2, aiming for better form and slightly longer hold times. Pay attention to your breath and proper alignment.

Week 4: Full-Body Wellness

Day 22-28:

Continue repeating the exercises from previous weeks, adjusting the intensity to your comfort level. Focus on fluid movements and maintaining good posture.

Day 29-30:

Repeat the entire program from Week 4, emphasizing quality over quantity. Perform each exercise mindfully and with intention.

Remember to listen to your body and never force any movement. These gentle exercises are meant to improve your overall well-being, flexibility, and balance. If you experience discomfort or pain, stop the exercise and consult with a healthcare professional.

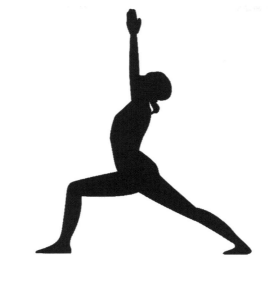

Illustrated
Exercises
for Wall Pilates

Wall Roll Down

Step 1

Step 2

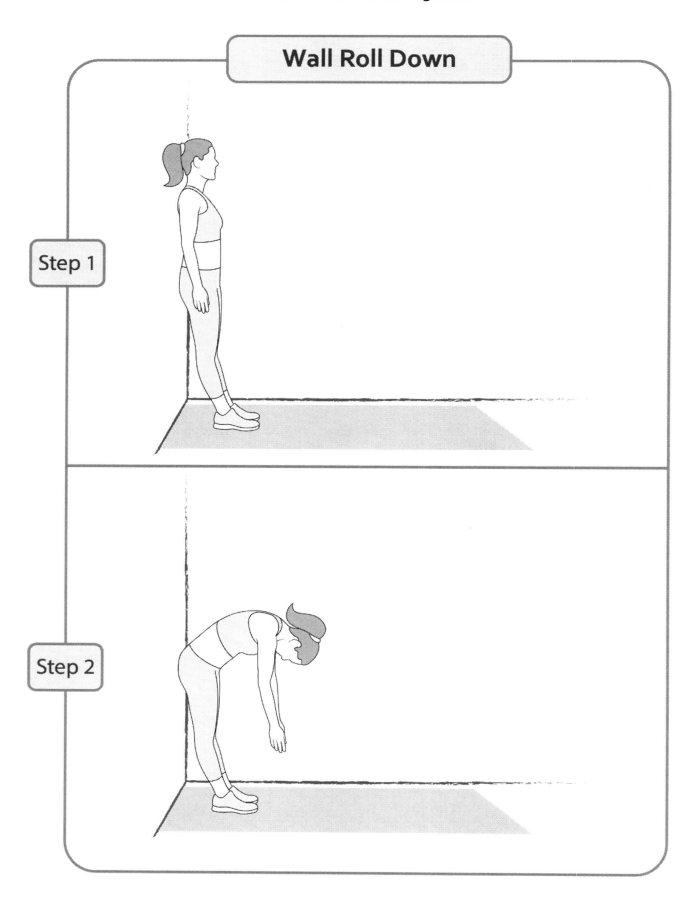

Wall Roll Down

Enhance Spinal Flexibility and Core Engagement

The Wall Roll Down is a foundational Pilates movement that combines spinal articulation with core engagement. This exercise promotes flexibility in the spine, stretches the hamstrings, and strengthens the core's muscles. By utilizing the support of a wall, you can focus on the sequential movement of each vertebra, promoting better body awareness and posture.

Instructions:

1. Stand with your back against a clear wall space, feet hip-width apart, and a few inches away from the wall.
2. Inhale deeply, lengthening your spine as you do.
3. Exhale as you begin the movement, slowly tucking your chin to your chest and initiating a sequential roll down of your spine.
4. Roll down one vertebra at a time, letting each touch the wall gradually, creating a rounded shape with your upper body.
5. Inhale deeply at the bottom of the movement while keeping your core engaged.
6. Exhale to reverse the movement, initiating the roll-up from your lower abdominals.
7. Stack each vertebra back up the wall, maintaining control and alignment.
8. Once fully upright, stand tall and inhale to lengthen your spine.

Tips:

- *Perform the movement in a deliberate and controlled manner, prioritizing alignment over speed.*
- *Keep your knees slightly bent throughout the exercise to protect your lower back and hamstrings.*
- *Visualize each vertebra touching the wall as you roll down and roll up.*
- *Maintain core engagement throughout to ensure stability and proper form.*
- *Avoid forcing your body into a deep stretch; always work within your comfortable range of motion.*
- *Incorporate breath awareness: exhale during the roll-down and inhale during the roll-up.*
- *Start with a small number of repetitions and gradually increase as your familiarity with the exercise grows.*

The Wall Roll Down exercise can be an excellent addition to your routine, aiding in enhancing spinal flexibility, strengthening the core, and refining body coordination.

Wall Squats

Step 1

Step 2

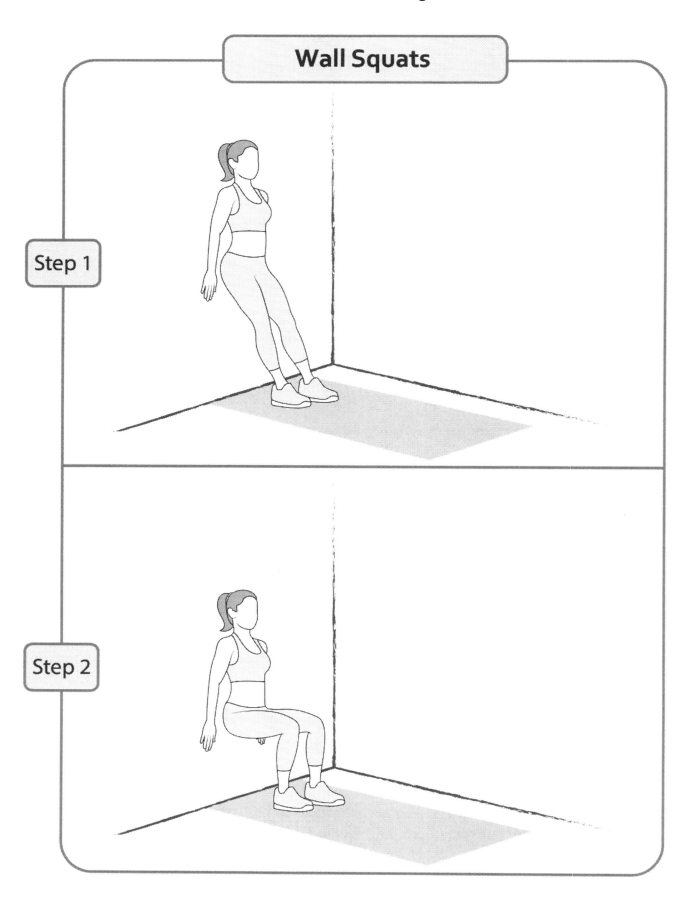

Wall Squats

Strengthen Lower Body and Improve Posture

Wall Squats are an effective lower-body exercise that engages your quads, hamstrings, and glutes while promoting proper posture. By using the wall for support, this exercise encourages correct alignment and controlled movement. It's an ideal option for building lower body strength without putting excessive strain on your knees or lower back.

Instructions:

1. Stand with your back against the wall, feet about hip-width apart, and a few inches away from the wall.
2. Engage your core by gently pulling your navel toward your spine.
3. Slide down the wall by bending your knees, as if you were sitting on an imaginary chair.
4. Lower yourself until your thighs are parallel to the ground, or as far down as your comfort allows.
5. Ensure your knees are directly above your ankles and tracking over your toes.
6. Press through your heels to stand back up, extending your legs.
7. Repeat the squat motion for the desired number of repetitions.

Tips:

- *Keep your spine against the wall and maintain proper posture throughout the movement.*
- *Focus on pushing your hips back and down as you lower yourself into the squat position.*
- *Avoid letting your knees' position go past your toes' to prevent unnecessary strain on your knees.*
- *Keep your weight in your heels and engage your glutes as you rise back up.*
- *Start with a moderate range of motion and gradually deepen the squat as your strength increases.*
- *Incorporate controlled breathing: inhale as you lower down and exhale as you stand back up.*
- *If you have any knee or lower back issues, consult a fitness professional before attempting this exercise.*

Wall Squats can contribute to improved lower body strength, functional movement, and better posture over time.

Wall Angel

Step 1

Step 2

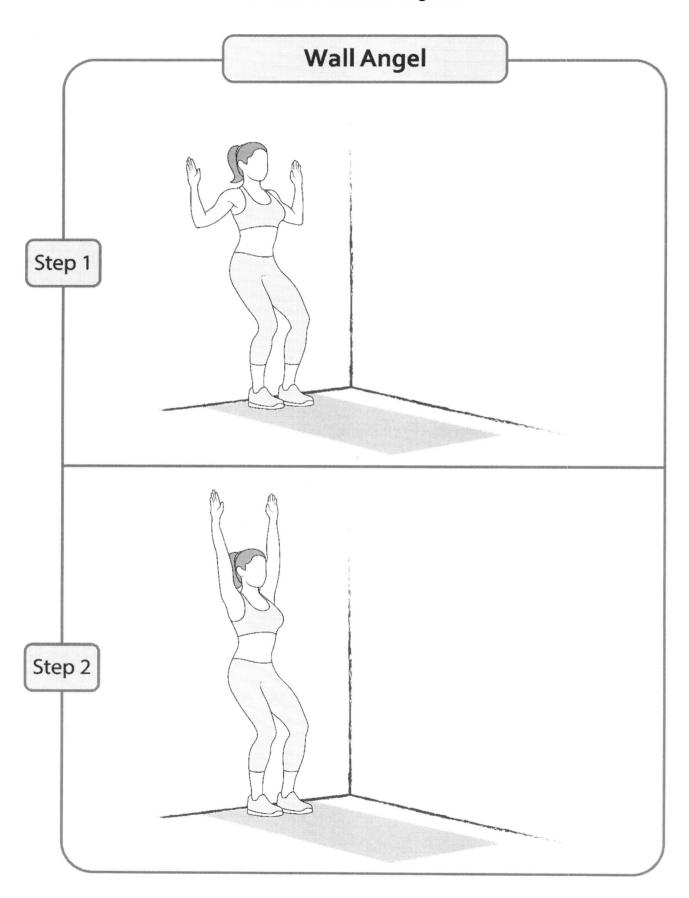

Wall Angel

Improve Shoulder Mobility and Posture

The Wall Angel is a movement that helps improve shoulder mobility and strengthen the muscles responsible for maintaining proper posture. By performing this exercise against a wall, you engage the muscles that support your spine and shoulders, enhancing body awareness and alignment.

Instructions:

1. Stand with your back against a wall, feet hip-width apart, and a slight distance from the wall.
2. Gently press your lower back against the wall, maintaining a neutral spine.
3. Bend your elbows at a 90-degree angle, and raise your arms to shoulder height, pressing your forearms against the wall.
4. Slowly slide your arms upward along the wall, extending your elbows as you raise your arms overhead.
5. Keep your forearms and hands in contact with the wall at all times.
6. Once your arms are fully extended overhead, reverse the movement by sliding your arms back down to the starting position.
7. Maintain engagement in your core muscles throughout the movement.

Tips:

- *Keep your wrists, elbows, and shoulders in alignment as you slide your arms.*
- *Focus on a controlled and fluid motion, avoiding any jerky movements.*
- *Keep your shoulders relaxed and away from your ears during the entire exercise.*
- *If you find it difficult to keep your lower back against the wall, perform a small pelvic tilt to engage your core.*
- *Breathe naturally during the movement: inhale as you slide up and exhale as you slide down.*
- *Start with a smaller range of motion and gradually work toward raising your arms fully overhead.*

The Wall Angel exercise can contribute to improved shoulder mobility, posture awareness, and overall upper body strength.

Wall Bridge

Step 1

Step 2

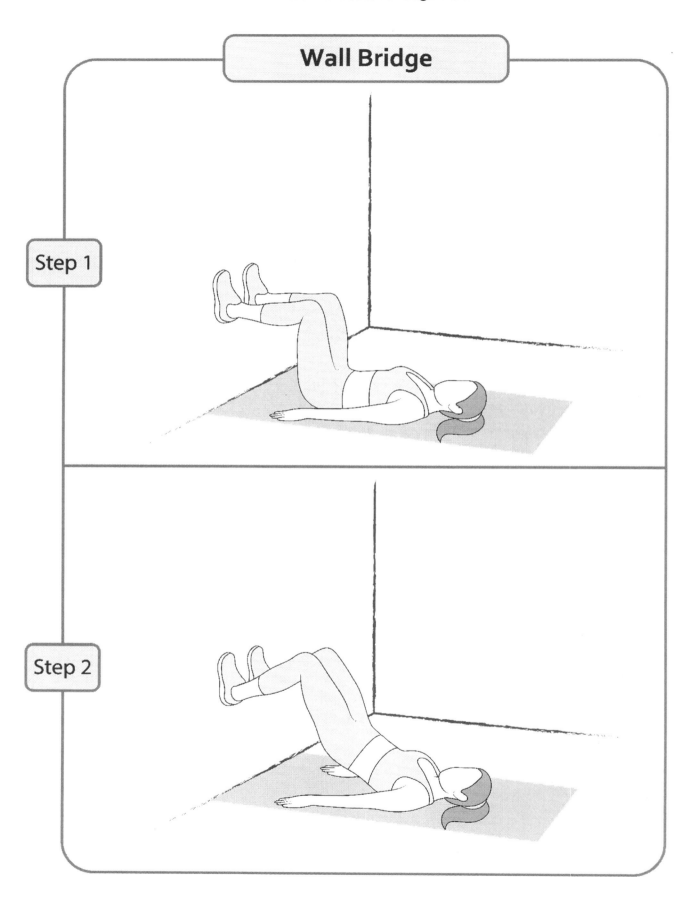

Wall Bridge

Strengthen Glutes and Hamstrings

The Wall Bridge is a targeted movement that engages your glutes and hamstrings while improving hip stability. Using the support of the wall, this exercise allows you to focus on controlled lifting and lowering of your hips, promoting proper form and muscle activation.

Instructions:

1. Lie on your back with your hips close to the wall and your feet hip-width apart.
2. Place your feet flat against the wall, knees bent at a 90-degree angle.
3. Extend your arms by your sides, palms facing down, for stability.
4. Engage your core by gently pulling your navel toward your spine.
5. Press your feet into the wall as you lift your hips off the floor, creating a diagonal line from your shoulders to your knees.
6. Squeeze your glutes at the top of the bridge to engage your hip muscles.
7. Lower your hips back down with control, maintaining engagement in your glutes and hamstrings.
8. Repeat the movement for the desired number of repetitions.

Tips:

- *Keep your feet hip-width apart and ensure your knees stay aligned with your feet.*
- *Maintain a neutral spine throughout the movement, avoiding arching or flattening your lower back.*
- *Press evenly through your feet into the wall to engage both sides of your glutes.*
- *Breathe naturally: inhale as you lower your hips and exhale as you lift them.*
- *Focus on lifting your hips with control, rather than using momentum.*
- *Start with a small number of repetitions and gradually increase as your strength improves.*

The Wall Bridge exercise can be an effective addition to your routine for enhancing lower body strength and stability.

Wall Plank

Step 1

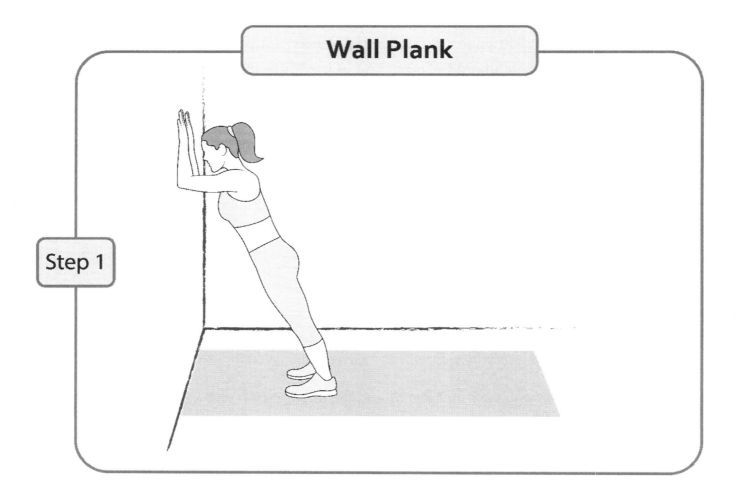

Wall Plank

Strengthen Core and Upper Body

The Wall Plank is a variation of the traditional plank that engages your core muscles while also targeting your upper body strength. By using the wall as support, this exercise allows you to focus on maintaining proper alignment and stability throughout your entire body.

Instructions:

1. Stand facing the wall and place your hands against it at shoulder height, slightly wider than shoulder-width apart.
2. Step your feet back, keeping your body in a straight line from head to heels.
3. Engage your core muscles by pulling your navel toward your spine.
4. Press your hands into the wall, creating tension in your shoulders and activating your chest and triceps.
5. Keep your body in a plank position, with your hips neither lifted nor drooping.
6. Hold the position for the desired duration, aiming for at least 20-30 seconds to start.

Tips:

- *Focus on maintaining a neutral spine, keeping your head aligned with your back.*
- *Engage your glutes to help stabilize your hips and prevent drooping.*
- *Keep your core muscles activated throughout the exercise.*
- *Press firmly through your hands, creating a strong connection with the wall.*
- *Breathe steadily and avoid holding your breath.*
- *As you become more comfortable, gradually increase the duration of the hold.*
- *If the wall plank feels too challenging, you can modify the exercise by performing it on your knees or with your hands placed slightly higher on the wall.*

The Wall Plank can be a valuable addition to your routine for building core strength, improving posture, and enhancing upper body stability.

Wall Side Leg Lifts

Step 1

Step 2

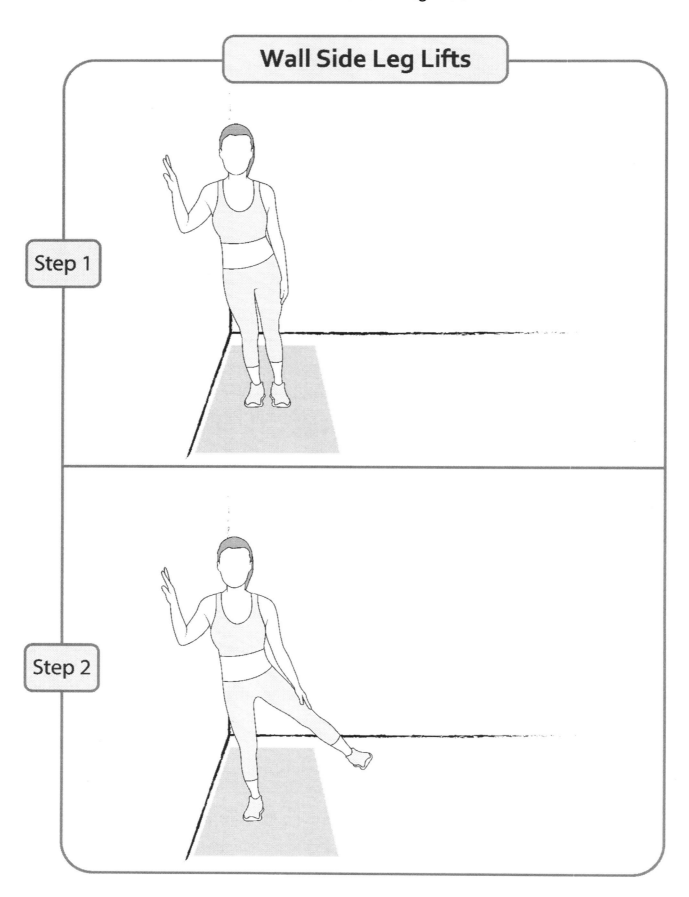

Wall Side Leg Lifts

Activate Hip Abductors and Improve Balance

Wall Side Leg Lifts are designed to activate your hip abductor muscles and improve balance. Using the support of the wall allows you to focus on controlled leg lifts, targeting the muscles responsible for moving your leg away from your body's midline.

Instructions:

1. Stand sideways to the wall, placing your hand on the wall for support.
2. Engage your core by gently pulling your navel toward your spine.
3. Lift one of your legs to the side, keeping it straight or with a slight bend in the knee.
4. Lift the leg to a comfortable height while maintaining balance and stability.
5. Lower your leg back down with control, but don't let it touch the ground.
6. Repeat the movement for the desired number of repetitions on one side.
7. Switch sides and perform the exercise with the opposite leg.

Tips:

- *Focus on keeping your upper body stable and avoid leaning toward the wall.*
- *Keep your core engaged to maintain proper alignment and balance.*
- *Keep the movement controlled, using your hip abductor muscles to lift the leg.*
- *Breathe naturally throughout the exercise.*
- *Start with a small number of repetitions and gradually increase as your strength and balance improve.*
- *For an added challenge, try performing the leg lifts without the support of the wall.*
- *If you have any concerns about balance or form, consider using a chair or support for balance.*

Wall Side Leg Lifts can be a beneficial way to strengthen hip abductors and enhance overall lower body stability.

Wall Teaser

Step 1

Step 2

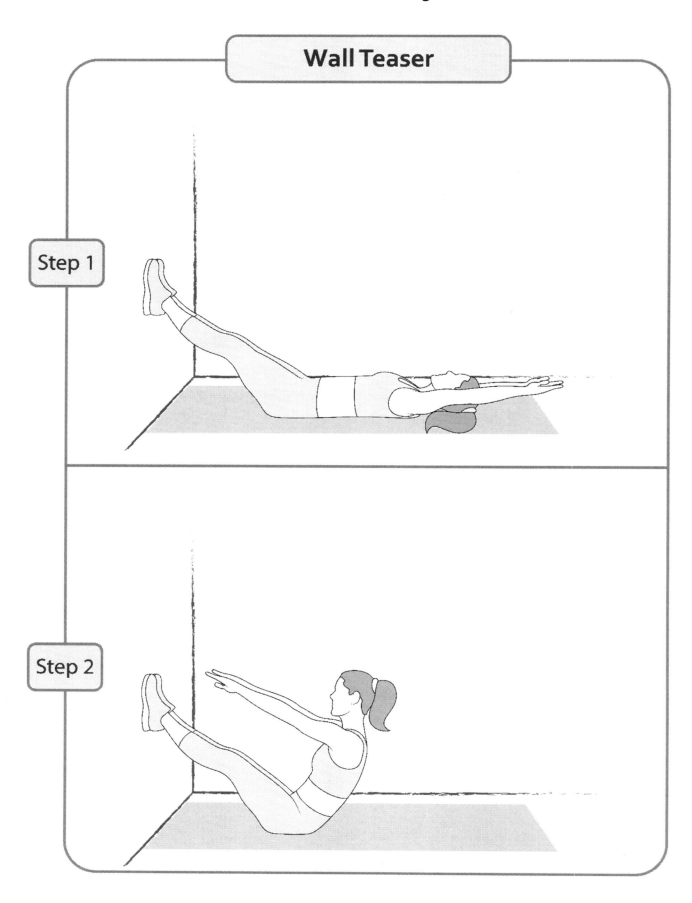

Wall Teaser

Enhance Core Strength and Spinal Mobility

The Wall Teaser is a challenging Pilates movement that focuses on strengthening your core muscles while promoting spinal mobility. By utilizing the wall as a guide, you can enhance your control and alignment during the movement. This exercise engages various muscle groups and encourages body awareness.

Instructions:

1. Sit on the floor facing the wall, with your knees bent and your feet flat against the wall.
2. Lean back slightly, engaging your core muscles.
3. Lift your feet off the floor and extend your legs, forming a "V" shape with your body.
4. Reach your arms forward, parallel to the ground, and press your palms against the wall.
5. Inhale deeply, and as you exhale, begin to round your spine and roll down one vertebra at a time.
6. Continue rolling back until your lower back touches the floor.
7. Inhale at the bottom of the movement, and as you exhale, initiate the roll-up.
8. Roll up with control, articulating your spine, and reaching your arms toward the wall.
9. Aim to return to the starting "V" position without letting your feet touch the ground.

Tips:

- *Keep your core engaged throughout the movement to control the descent and ascent.*
- *Maintain a steady breath pattern: exhale during the roll-down and inhale during the roll-up.*
- *Focus on the quality of movement rather than speed.*
- *If you have tight hamstrings, bend your knees slightly during the "V" position.*
- *Start with a smaller range of motion and gradually increase as you build strength and flexibility.*
- *Avoid using momentum; rely on your core muscles for the movement.*
- *If you find the exercise challenging, practice the motion without extending your legs fully.*

The Wall Teaser is a dynamic way to enhance core strength and spinal flexibility. Always prioritize proper form and listen to your body.

Wall Single Leg Stretch

Step 1

Step 2

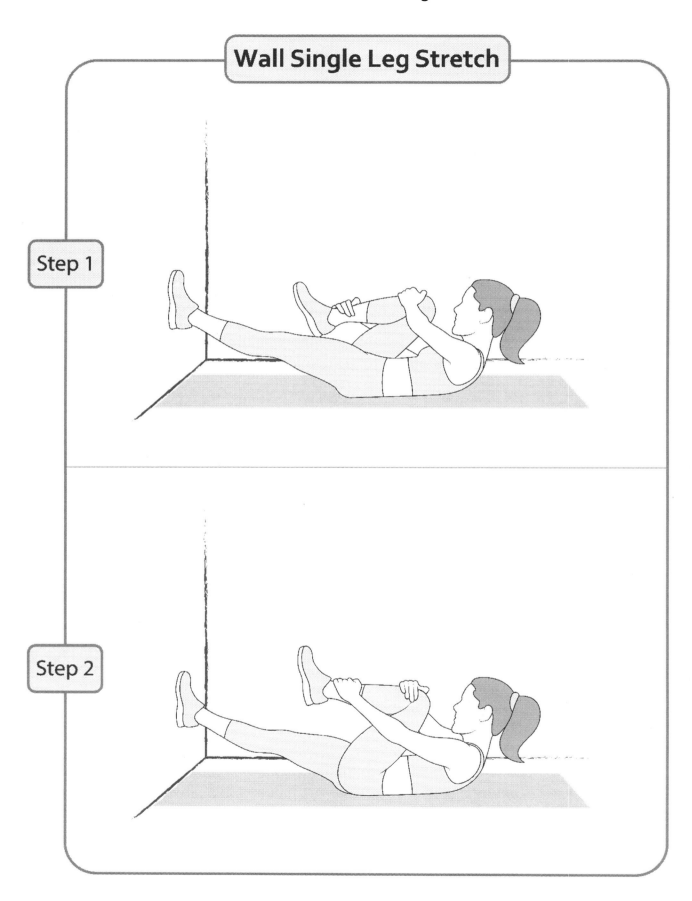

Wall Single Leg Stretch

Strengthen Core and Improve Hip Flexibility

The Wall Single Leg Stretch is designed to strengthen your core muscles while enhancing hip flexibility and control. Using the wall as support, this exercise allows you to focus on maintaining stability and alignment as you perform alternating leg movements.

Instructions:

1. Lie on your back with your hips close to the wall and your legs extended up the wall.
2. Press your lower back into the floor and engage your core muscles.
3. Lift your head, neck, and shoulders off the ground.
4. Extend your right leg up the wall while keeping your left leg hovering slightly above the ground.
5. Inhale as you switch legs, bringing your left leg up the wall and your right leg hovering.
6. Simultaneously, exhale and lift your upper body higher while bringing your opposite elbow toward your bent knee.
7. Continue alternating legs while coordinating the upper body movement.

Tips:

- *Keep your lower back pressed into the floor to avoid arching.*
- *Maintain a steady breathing pattern: exhale during the upper body movement and inhale during the leg switch.*
- *Focus on engaging your core to lift your upper body, avoiding straining your neck.*
- *Keep your extended leg straight and toes pointing upward.*
- *Start with a slower pace to establish proper form and coordination.*
- *Aim for controlled and fluid movements rather than rushing.*
- *Gradually increase the number of repetitions as you build strength and coordination.*

The Wall Single Leg Stretch is effective for building core strength, enhancing hip flexibility, and improving coordination. As with any exercise, perform it mindfully and within your comfort level.

Wall Pike

Step 1

Step 2

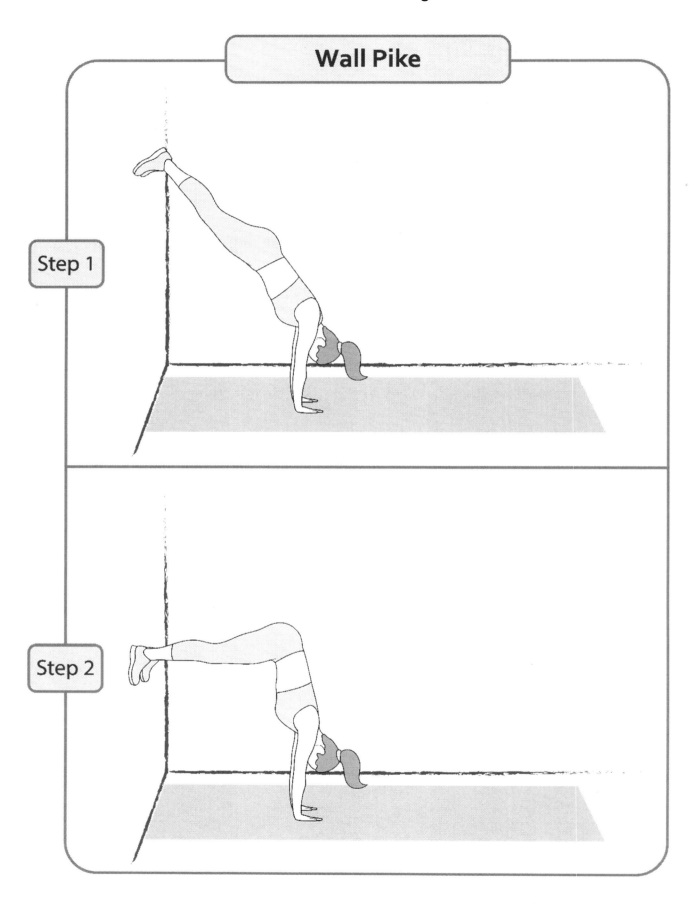

Wall Pike

Strengthen Core and Shoulders

The Wall Pike is a challenging movement that targets your core muscles while also engaging your shoulders and upper body. This exercise, utilizing the wall for support, encourages controlled and coordinated movement, enhancing core strength and shoulder stability.

Instructions:

1. Begin in a high plank position with your hands on the floor and your feet against the wall.
2. Your body should form a straight line from head to heels.
3. Engage your core muscles by pulling your navel toward your spine.
4. Slowly walk your feet up the wall while lifting your hips toward the ceiling.
5. As you walk your feet higher, your body will form an inverted "V" shape.
6. Keep your arms and shoulders engaged to maintain stability.
7. Hold the pike position briefly, feeling the stretch in your hamstrings and the engagement in your core and shoulders.
8. Slowly walk your feet back down to the starting plank position.

Tips:

- *Maintain a strong plank position with your core engaged throughout the movement.*
- *Focus on pressing through your hands to maintain stability and prevent wrist discomfort.*
- *Keep your neck in line with your spine; avoid looking up or down.*
- *Breathe naturally during the exercise, but avoid holding your breath.*
- *Start with a smaller pike angle and gradually work toward a deeper pike position.*
- *If you're new to this exercise, practice with small movements before attempting a full pike.*

The Wall Pike exercise is effective for strengthening your core, improving shoulder stability, and enhancing overall body control.

Wall Scissor

Step 1

Step 2

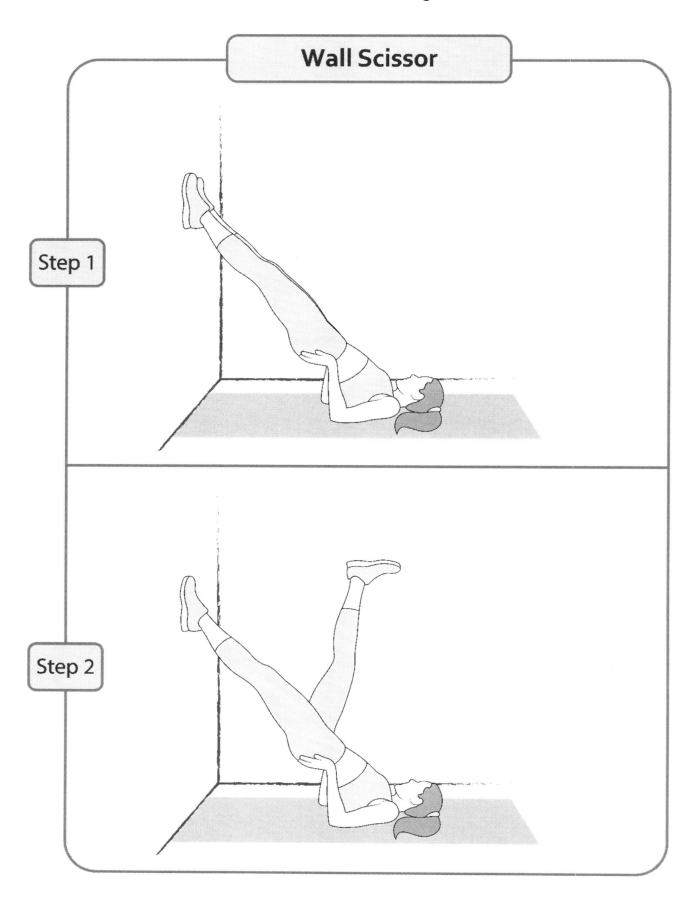

Wall Scissor

Engage Core and Improve Leg Flexibility

The Wall Scissor is a dynamic movement that engages your core muscles while enhancing leg flexibility. This exercise, performed against a wall, allows you to focus on controlled leg movements while maintaining stability and alignment.

Instructions:

1. Lie on your back with your hips close to the wall and your legs extended up the wall.
2. Press your lower back into the floor and engage your core muscles.
3. Place your hands by your sides for support.
4. Lower one leg toward the floor, keeping it straight or with a slight bend in the knee.
5. As you lower one leg, simultaneously raise the other leg toward the ceiling.
6. Keep your core engaged to stabilize your pelvis and lower back.
7. Alternate between lowering and raising your legs in a scissor-like motion.

Tips:

- *Maintain a neutral spine and avoid arching your lower back.*
- *Focus on controlled and deliberate leg movements.*
- *Keep your core engaged to prevent excessive movement in your pelvis.*
- *Breathe naturally throughout the exercise.*
- *Keep your legs straight and your toes pointed throughout the scissor motion.*
- *Start with a smaller range of motion and gradually increase as your flexibility and strength improve.*

The Wall Scissor is an effective way to engage your core and improve leg flexibility.

Wall Push-Ups

Step 1

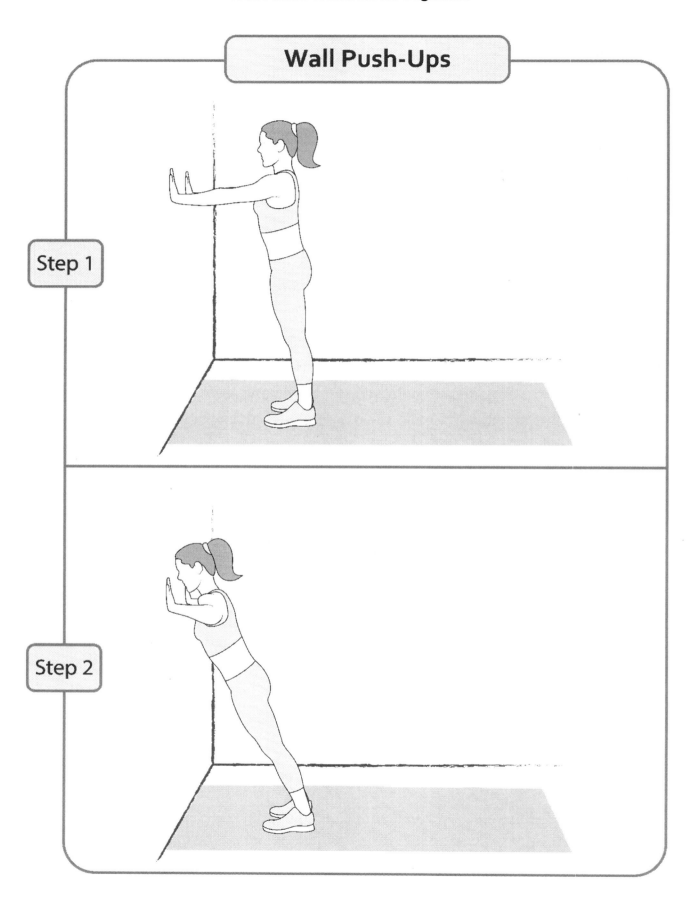

Step 2

Wall Push-Ups

Strengthen Upper Body and Core

Wall Push-Ups are a modified version of the traditional push-up that targets your upper body muscles while engaging your core. By using the wall as support, you can adjust the intensity of the movement to your fitness level, making it a great option for building upper body strength.

Instructions:

1. Stand facing the wall at arms' length away, and place your hands on the wall at shoulder height, slightly wider than shoulder-width apart.
2. Step back a comfortable distance from the wall while keeping your body in a straight line from head to heels.
3. Engage your core muscles by pulling your navel toward your spine.
4. Inhale as you bend your elbows, lowering your chest toward the wall.
5. Exhale as you push through your palms, extending your elbows and returning to the starting position.
6. Focus on maintaining a straight line from head to heels throughout the movement.
7. Repeat the push-up motion for the desired number of repetitions.

Tips:

- *Keep your core engaged to maintain stability and prevent your lower back from drooping.*
- *Ensure your wrists are aligned with your shoulders and your hands are pressing evenly on the wall.*
- *Maintain a controlled pace, avoiding fast or jerky movements.*
- *Breathe naturally during the exercise, exhaling as you push away from the wall.*
- *If you find the exercise challenging, step closer to the wall to reduce the angle of your body.*
- *Progress to a greater distance from the wall as your strength increases.*

Wall Push-Ups are an effective way to build upper body strength and engage your core. As with any exercise, perform it with proper form and consult a fitness professional if you're new to this exercise or have any concerns.

Wall Lunge Stretch

Step 1

Step 2

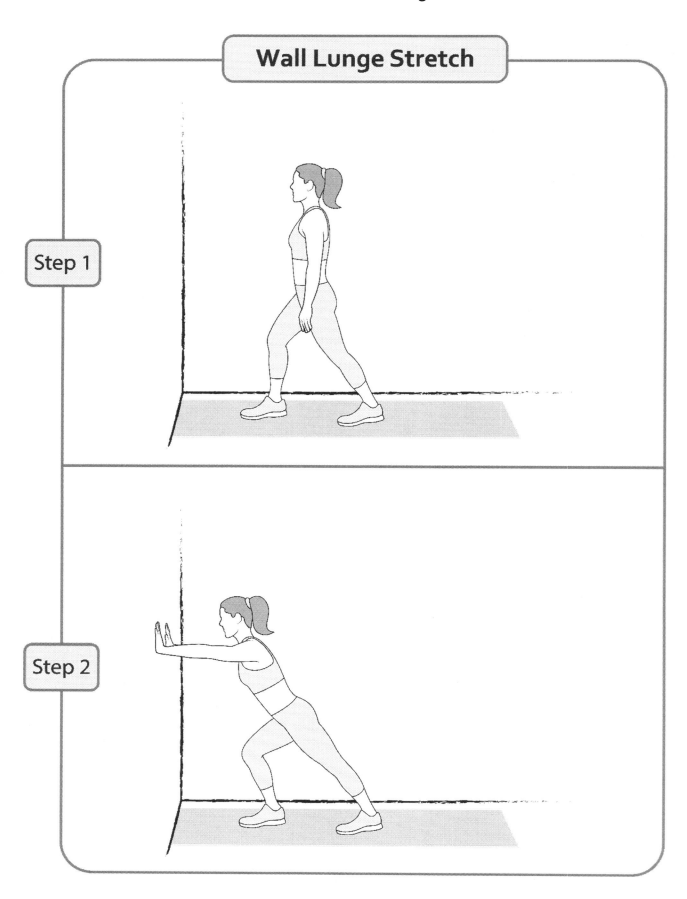

Wall Lunge Stretch

Improve Lower Body Flexibility

The Wall Lunge Stretch is designed to improve lower body flexibility, particularly in the hip flexors and quadriceps. By utilizing the support of the wall, you can maintain proper alignment and deepen the stretch safely.

Instructions:

1. Stand facing the wall, about an arm's length away.
2. Place your hands on the wall at shoulder height for support.
3. Step one foot forward, keeping a comfortable distance between your feet.
4. Bend your front knee and lower your back knee toward the floor, as if you were moving into a lunge position.
5. Press your foot against the wall, allowing your back hip to gently lean toward the wall.
6. Feel the stretch along the front of your hip and thigh.
7. Hold the stretch for the desired duration, focusing on relaxing and breathing.

Tips:

- *Keep your front knee aligned with your ankle, preventing it from going past your toes.*
- *Engage your core to maintain proper posture and alignment throughout the stretch.*
- *Ensure your back knee is hovering just above the ground to avoid excess pressure on the knee joint.*
- *Breathe deeply and steadily, inhaling as you relax into the stretch.*
- *If you experience discomfort, adjust the depth of the lunge or the distance from the wall.*
- *To deepen the stretch, gently press your pelvis forward and upward toward the wall.*

The Wall Lunge Stretch is an effective way to enhance lower body flexibility and improve hip mobility.

Wall Hip Abduction

Step 1

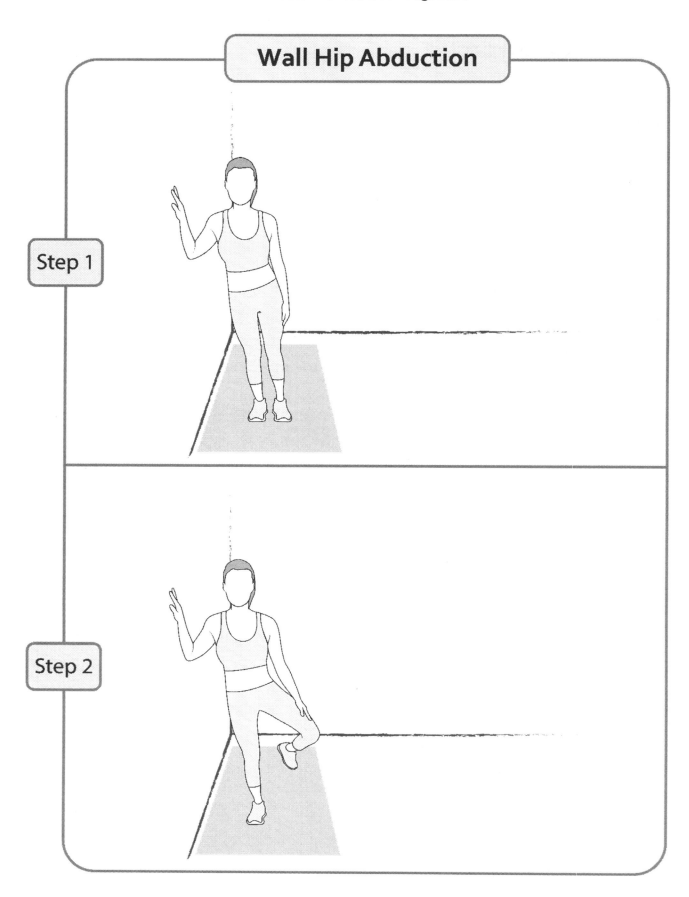

Step 2

Wall Hip Abduction

Strengthen Hip Muscles and Improve Stability

The Wall Hip Abduction targets the hip abductor muscles, which are responsible for moving your leg away from your body's midline. By using the wall for support, this exercise allows you to focus on controlled movements and engage the muscles that contribute to overall lower body stability.

Instructions:

1. Stand sideways to the wall, placing your hand on it for support.
2. Engage your core muscles by gently pulling your navel toward your spine.
3. Lift your outer leg to the side, keeping it straight or with a slight bend in the knee.
4. Lift the leg to a comfortable height while maintaining balance and stability.
5. Lower your leg back down with control, but don't let it touch the ground.
6. Repeat the movement for the desired number of repetitions on one side.
7. Switch sides and perform the exercise with the opposite leg.

Tips:

- *Focus on keeping your upper body stable and avoid leaning toward the wall.*
- *Keep your core engaged to maintain proper alignment and balance.*
- *Keep the movement controlled, using your hip abductor muscles to lift the leg.*
- *Breathe naturally throughout the exercise.*
- *Start with a small number of repetitions and gradually increase as your strength and balance improve.*
- *For an added challenge, try performing the leg lifts without the support of the wall.*
- *If you have any concerns about balance or form, consider using a chair or support for balance.*

The Wall Hip Abduction is a beneficial way to strengthen hip abductors and enhance overall lower body stability.

Wall Side Plank

Step 1

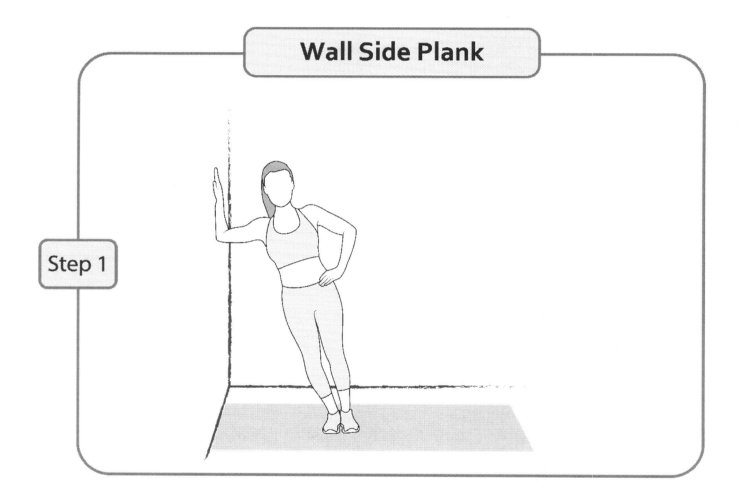

Wall Side Plank

Enhance Core and Side Body Strength

The Wall Side Plank is a variation of the traditional side plank that focuses on strengthening the core muscles and the muscles along the side of your body. Using the wall for support, this exercise allows you to maintain proper alignment and engage the muscles responsible for stabilizing your torso.

Instructions:

1. Stand sideways against the wall at arms' length
2. Raise your arm at shoulder height towards the wall and bend it so that the palm is pointing upward.
3. Align your feet and hips, creating a straight line from head to heels.
4. Put your elbow against the wall.
5. Ensure your body remains in a straight line without drooping or hiking your hips.
6. Hold the side plank for the desired duration, maintaining proper alignment.
7. Repeat the exercise on the opposite side.

Tips:

- *Focus on maintaining a straight line from your head to your heels.*
- *Engage your core muscles to stabilize your torso throughout the exercise.*
- *Avoid letting your hips drop or your shoulders collapse.*
- *Breathe naturally; do not hold your breath.*
- *Gradually increase the duration of the hold as your strength improves.*
- *If you have any shoulder issues, consult a fitness professional before attempting this exercise.*

The Wall Side Plank is an effective way to build core strength and engage the muscles along the side of your body.

Wall Corkscrew

Step 1

Step 2

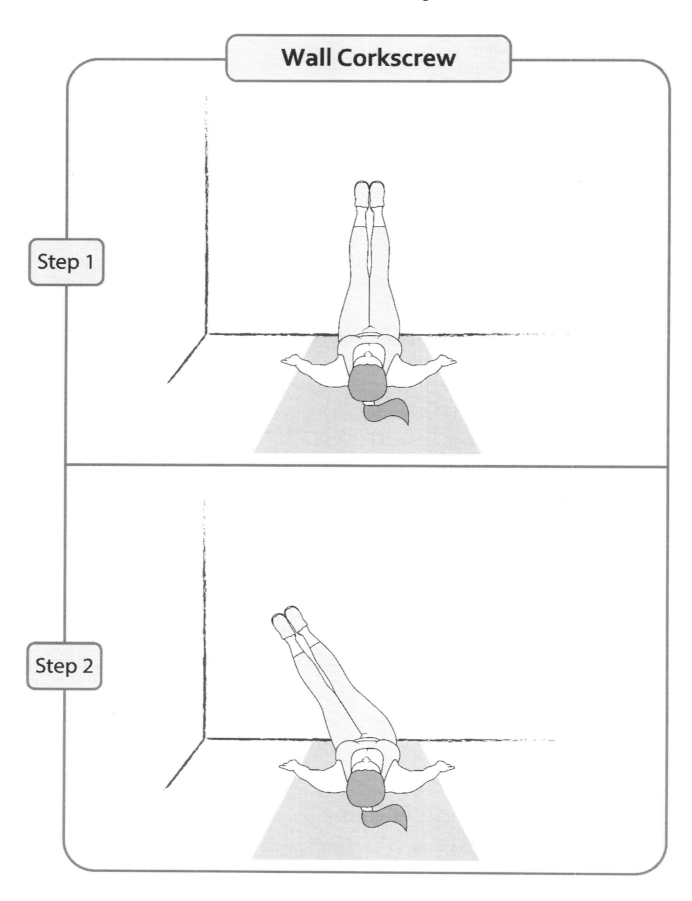

Wall Corkscrew

Enhance Spinal Mobility and Core Engagement

The Wall Corkscrew is a dynamic Pilates movement that focuses on improving spinal mobility while engaging the core muscles. By utilizing the wall as a guide, this exercise encourages controlled movement and sequential articulation of the spine. It targets various muscle groups and promotes body awareness.

Instructions:

1. Lie on your back with your hips close to the wall and your legs extended up the wall.
2. Press your lower back into the floor and engage your core muscles.
3. Extend your arms out to the sides, palms facing down, for stability.
4. Inhale deeply to prepare, and as you exhale, begin to lower your legs to one side.
5. Lower your legs as far as you can while maintaining control and engagement in your core.
6. Inhale as you start to lift your legs back up, bringing them to the center.
7. Exhale and lower your legs to the opposite side, keeping the movement controlled.
8. Inhale as you lift your legs back up to the center.
9. Continue alternating sides, moving in a fluid and controlled manner.

Tips:

- *Keep your shoulders and arms connected to the floor for stability.*
- *Engage your core muscles throughout the movement to protect your lower back.*
- *Focus on maintaining a consistent breath pattern: exhale during the lowering phase and inhale during the lifting phase.*
- *Move through the exercise with control, avoiding any sudden or jerky movements.*
- *Start with a small range of motion and gradually increase as your flexibility and strength improve.*
- *Keep your legs straight and your feet flexed during the movement.*

The Wall Corkscrew can contribute to enhanced spinal mobility, core engagement, and body coordination.

Wall Roll Up

Step 1

Step 2

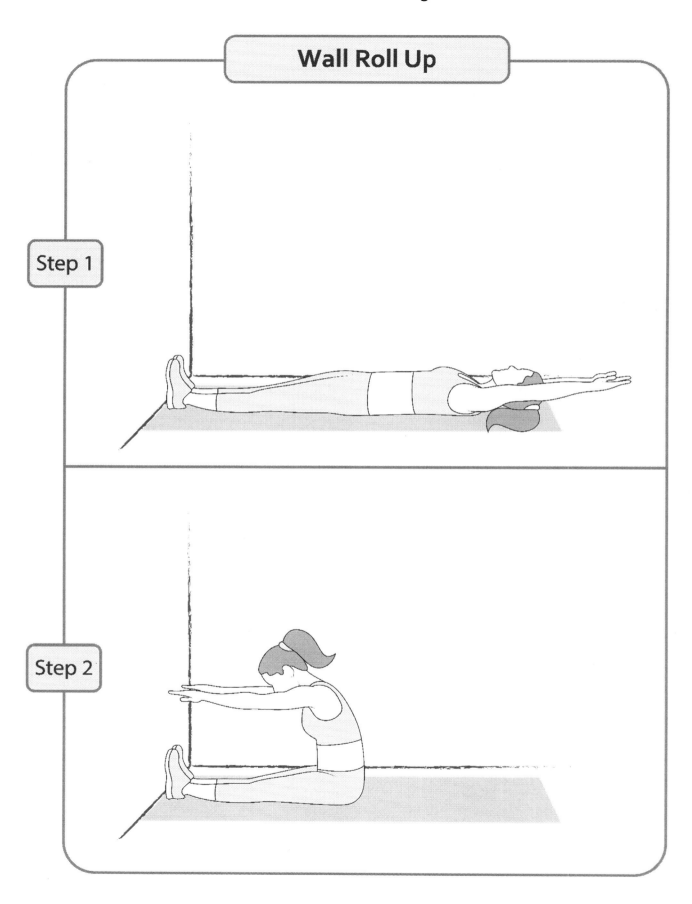

Wall Roll Up

Enhance Spinal Mobility and Core Strength

The Wall Roll Up is a Pilates movement that focuses on improving spinal mobility and engaging the core's muscles. Using the wall for support, this exercise guides you through a controlled movement that targets the entire length of the spine. It's an excellent way to promote flexibility, strength, and body awareness.

Instructions:

1. Sit on the floor facing the wall, with your legs extended and your feet against it.
2. Stretch your arms forward, parallel to the ground, and press your palms against the wall.
3. Inhale deeply to prepare, engaging your core muscles.
4. Exhale as you begin the movement, initiating a sequential roll down of your spine.
5. Slowly articulate your spine, lowering your torso toward the floor, one vertebra at a time.
6. As you roll down, maintain contact between your lower back and the floor.
7. Inhale deeply at the bottom of the movement while keeping your core engaged.
8. Exhale as you initiate the roll-up, engaging your abdominals to lift your torso.
9. Roll up through each vertebra, reaching your arms forward as you return to the starting position.

Tips:

- *Focus on controlled movement, segmentally rolling down and up through your spine.*
- *Engage your core muscles throughout the exercise to protect your lower back.*
- *Maintain a consistent breath pattern: exhale during the roll-down and inhale during the roll-up.*
- *Keep your shoulders relaxed and away from your ears.*
- *Visualize each vertebra as it touches the mat during the roll-down and lifts during the roll-up.*
- *Start with a smaller range of motion if flexibility is limited, and gradually increase as you progress.*

The Wall Roll Up can help enhance spinal mobility, strengthen the core's muscles, and improve body alignment.

Wall Arm Circles

Step 1

Step 2

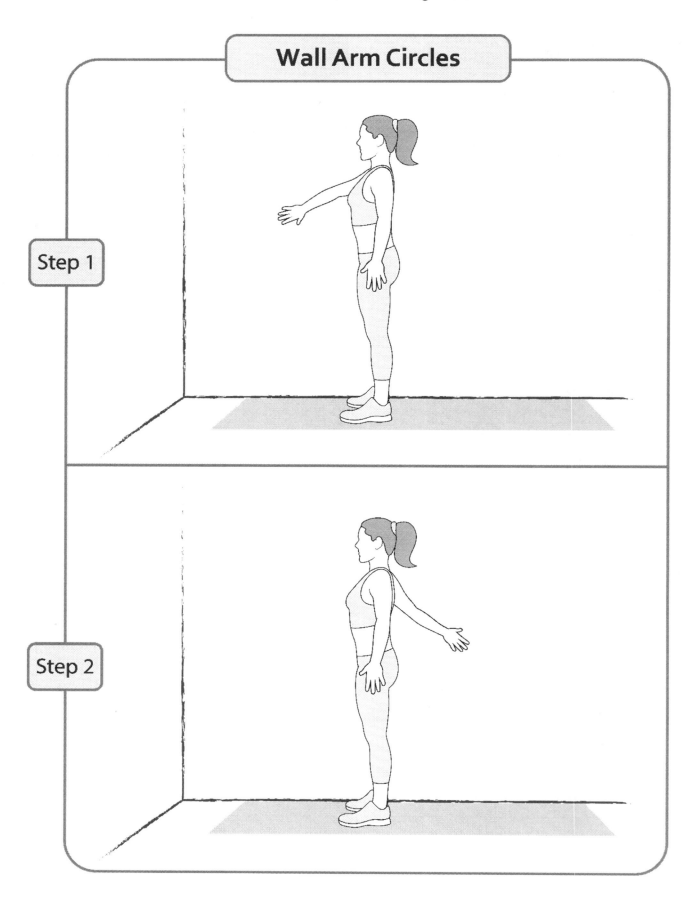

Wall Arm Circles

Improve Shoulder Mobility and Stability

Wall Arm Circles are designed to enhance shoulder mobility and stability while engaging the muscles of the upper body. By using the wall for support, this exercise allows you to focus on controlled movement and proper alignment of the shoulders.

Instructions:

1. Stand sideways to the wall, with your feet hip-width apart and your hands resting against the wall at shoulder height.
2. Press your palms into the wall while engaging your core muscles.
3. Keep a slight bend in your elbows as you initiate the movement.
4. Begin to make small circular motions with your arms against the wall.
5. Gradually increase the size of the circles, focusing on smooth and controlled movements.
6. Continue circling your arms for the desired number of repetitions or time.
7. Reverse the direction of the circles to work through the full range of motion.

Tips:

- *Maintain a stable core to prevent excessive arching or rounding of the lower back.*
- *Keep your shoulders relaxed and away from your ears throughout the exercise.*
- *Focus on controlled movements, avoiding jerky or abrupt motions.*
- *Breathe naturally during the exercise, inhaling and exhaling steadily.*
- *Engage your shoulder muscles to control the movement and maintain proper alignment.*
- *Gradually increase the size of the circles as your shoulder mobility improves.*
- *If you experience discomfort or strain, reduce the size of the circles or decrease the range of motion.*

Wall Arm Circles can be beneficial for improving shoulder mobility, enhancing upper body coordination, and promoting shoulder stability.

Wall Tricep Dips

Step 1

Step 2

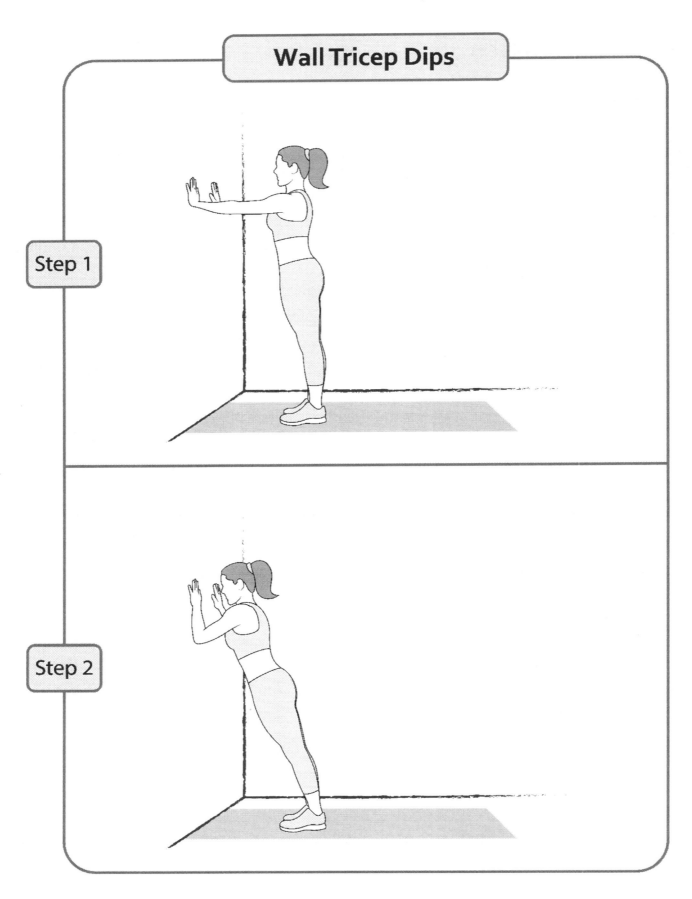

Wall Triceps Dips

Strengthen Triceps and Upper Body

Wall Triceps Dips target the triceps muscles while also engaging the muscles of the upper body and core. By using the wall for support, you can control the intensity of the exercise and focus on proper form. This exercise is effective for building strength in the back of the arms.

Instructions:

1. Stand facing a wall with your feet hip-width apart
2. Stand at an arm's length away from the wall.
3. Extend your arms straight in front of you, shoulder-width apart.
4. Place your palms flat against the wall, fingers pointing upward.
5. Inhale as you bend your elbows, lowering your body toward the wall.
6. Keep your body in a straight line from head to heels.
7. Exhale as you push against the wall, extending your arms fully.
8. Focus on engaging your triceps as you push.
9. Complete the desired number of repetitions.
10. A common starting point is 2-3 sets of 10-15 repetitions.

Tips:

* *Keep your core engaged to maintain proper alignment and stability.*
* *Focus on pressing through your palms to engage your triceps.*
* *Avoid letting your shoulders shrug up toward your ears; keep them relaxed.*
* *Breathe naturally throughout the exercise.*
* *As your strength improves, you can increase the angle for a greater challenge.*
* *Make sure your wrists are comfortable; consider adjusting your hand position if needed.*

Wall Triceps Dips are an effective way to strengthen the triceps and engage the upper body muscles.

Wall Push-Up with Leg Lift

Step 1

Step 2

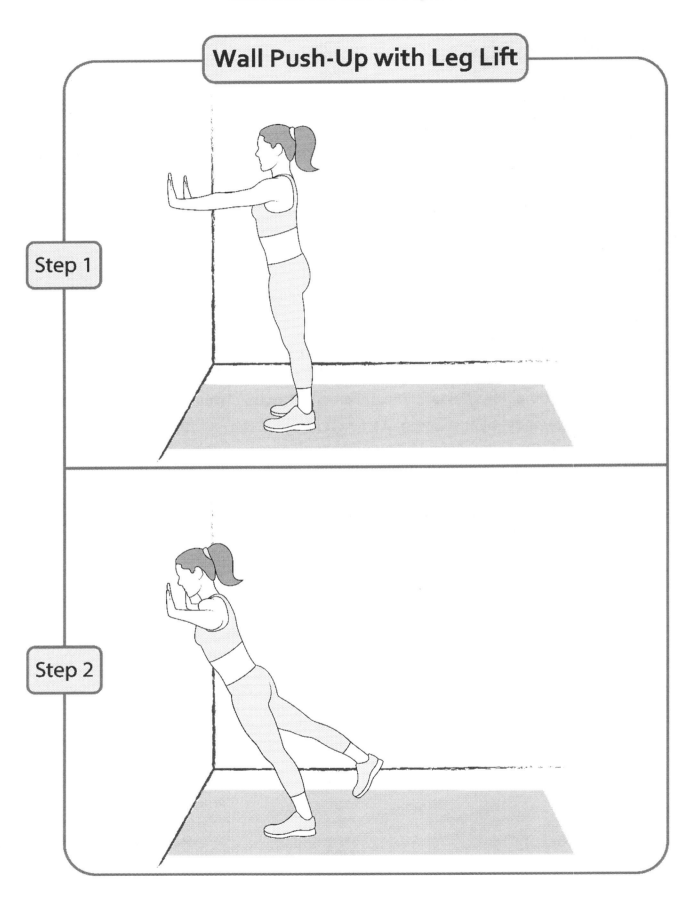

Wall Push-Up with Leg Lift

Engage Upper Body and Core Muscles

The Wall Push-Up with Leg Lift combines the benefits of a push-up with the engagement of the core and lower body. By using the wall for support, you can tailor the exercise to your fitness level and focus on upper body and core strength.

Instructions:

1. Stand facing the wall, about arms' length away.
2. Place your hands on the wall slightly wider than shoulder-width apart.
3. Step back, extending your legs and forming a diagonal line from head to heels.
4. Engage your core muscles by pulling your navel toward your spine.
5. Inhale as you bend your elbows, lowering your chest toward the wall.
6. As you exhale, push through your palms to extend your elbows and return to the starting position.
7. After completing a push-up, lift one leg slightly off the ground, engaging your glutes.
8. Lower the leg back down and perform another push-up.
9. Alternate lifting each leg after each push-up repetition.

Tips:

- *Keep your core engaged to maintain proper alignment and stability.*
- *Focus on pressing through your palms to engage your chest and triceps.*
- *Keep your body in a straight line throughout the exercise.*
- *Breathe naturally during the exercise.*
- *For added stability, engage your glutes as you lift each leg.*
- *Modify the exercise by performing push-ups without the leg lift if needed.*
- *Gradually increase the number of repetitions as your strength improves.*

The Wall Push-Up with Leg Lift is a compound movement that works the upper body and engages the core and lower body muscles.

Wall Reverse Plank

Step 1

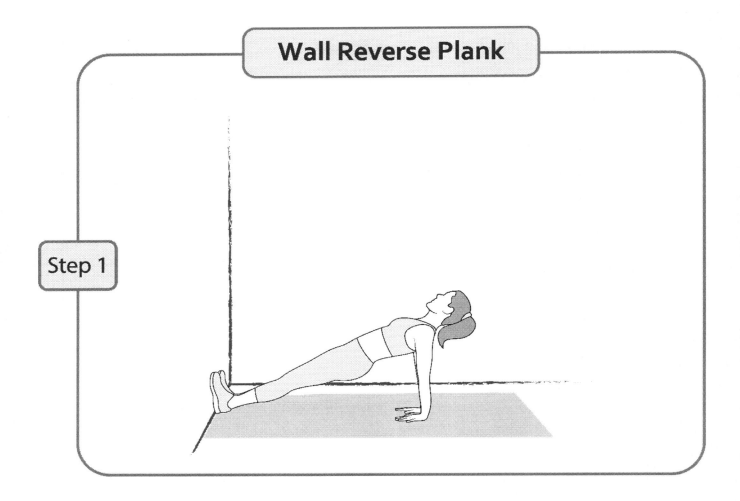

Wall Reverse Plank

Strengthen Upper Body and Core

The Wall Reverse Plank is a variation of the traditional plank that targets the upper body and engages the core muscles. By using the wall for support, this exercise allows you to focus on building strength in the shoulders, triceps, and core while improving overall stability.

Instructions:

1. Sit on the floor facing the wall, with your legs extended in front of you.
2. Place your hands on the floor behind you, fingers pointing toward the wall.
3. Press your palms and heels into the ground, lifting your hips off the floor.
4. Walk your feet forward, creating a diagonal line from your head to your heels.
5. Engage your core muscles by pulling your navel toward your spine.
6. Keep your body in a straight line, avoiding any drooping or lifting of the hips.
7. Hold the position for the desired duration, focusing on maintaining stability.

Tips:

- *Keep your shoulders away from your ears, and your chest should be open.*
- *Press through your palms and heels to engage your triceps and glutes.*
- *Maintain a steady breath pattern throughout the exercise.*
- *Focus on keeping your hips lifted and core engaged to prevent drooping.*
- *If the exercise is too challenging, start with your knees bent and feet flat on the floor.*
- *Gradually progress to the full reverse plank position as your strength improves.*

The Wall Reverse Plank is effective for building upper body and core strength, as well as enhancing stability.

Wall Torso Rotation

Step 1

Step 2

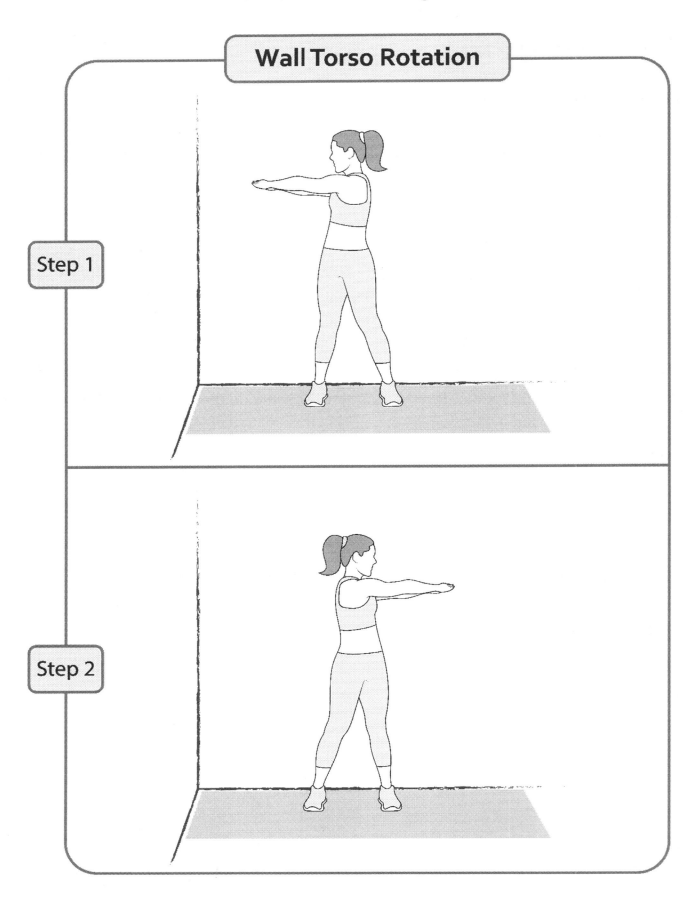

Wall Torso Rotation

Enhance Core and Oblique Strength

The Wall Torso Rotation is designed to engage the core muscles and target the obliques, which are the muscles along the sides of your abdomen. By using the wall for resistance, this exercise provides a controlled way to work on rotational strength and stability.

Instructions:

1. Stand facing the wall, about arms' length away.
2. Extend your arms forward, parallel to the ground, and press your palms against the wall.
3. Position your feet hip-width apart and engage your core muscles.
4. Slowly rotate your torso to one side, leading with your ribcage.
5. Keep your hips and legs facing forward while your upper body turns.
6. Inhale as you rotate to one side, and exhale as you return to the center.
7. Perform the rotation to the other side, leading with your ribcage again.
8. Continue alternating rotations for the desired number of repetitions.

Tips:

- *Keep your core engaged to maintain stability throughout the exercise.*
- *Focus on controlled rotation without using momentum.*
- *Breathe naturally during the movement, exhaling as you rotate.*
- *Keep your hips and legs stable, allowing only your upper body to move.*
- *Avoid tensing your neck and shoulders; keep them relaxed.*
- *Start with a smaller range of motion and gradually increase as you feel more comfortable.*
- *If the exercise feels too challenging, lessen the pressure against the wall.*

The Wall Torso Rotation is effective for engaging the oblique muscles and enhancing rotational strength.

Wall Mermaid Stretch

Step 1

Step 2

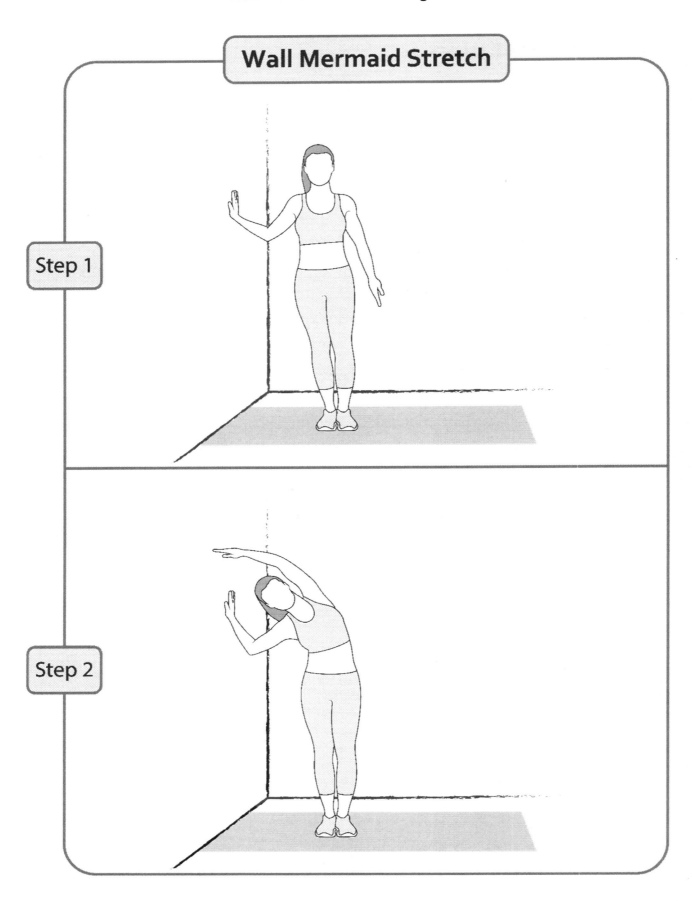

Wall Mermaid Stretch

Improve Side Body Flexibility

The Wall Mermaid Stretch is designed to enhance flexibility along the side of your body, particularly in the ribs and waist. By using the wall for support, you can maintain proper alignment and deepen the stretch effectively.

Instructions:

1. Stand sideways to the wall, placing your hand on the wall for support at shoulder height.
2. Extend the arm closer to the wall and press your palm against it.
3. Step your feet away from the wall, creating a diagonal line from your hand to your opposite foot.
4. Engage your core muscles to maintain proper posture.
5. Inhale deeply to lengthen your spine, and as you exhale, begin to lean your torso sideways.
6. Feel the stretch along the side of your body, from your fingertips down to your hip.
7. Hold the stretch for the desired duration while continuing to breathe.
8. Inhale as you return to an upright position.
9. Switch sides and repeat the stretch with the opposite arm and leg.

Tips:

- *Keep your hips aligned and avoid arching or leaning forward or backward.*
- *Engage your core muscles to support your spine during the stretch.*
- *Breathe deeply and steadily as you hold the stretch.*
- *Gently increase the stretch as you exhale and relax into it.*
- *Focus on maintaining length on both sides of your body while stretching.*
- *If you experience discomfort, reduce the depth of the stretch.*
- *Consult a fitness professional if you have any concerns about your form or flexibility.*

The Wall Mermaid Stretch is a beneficial way to improve side body flexibility and increase body awareness.

Wall Split Stretch

Step 1

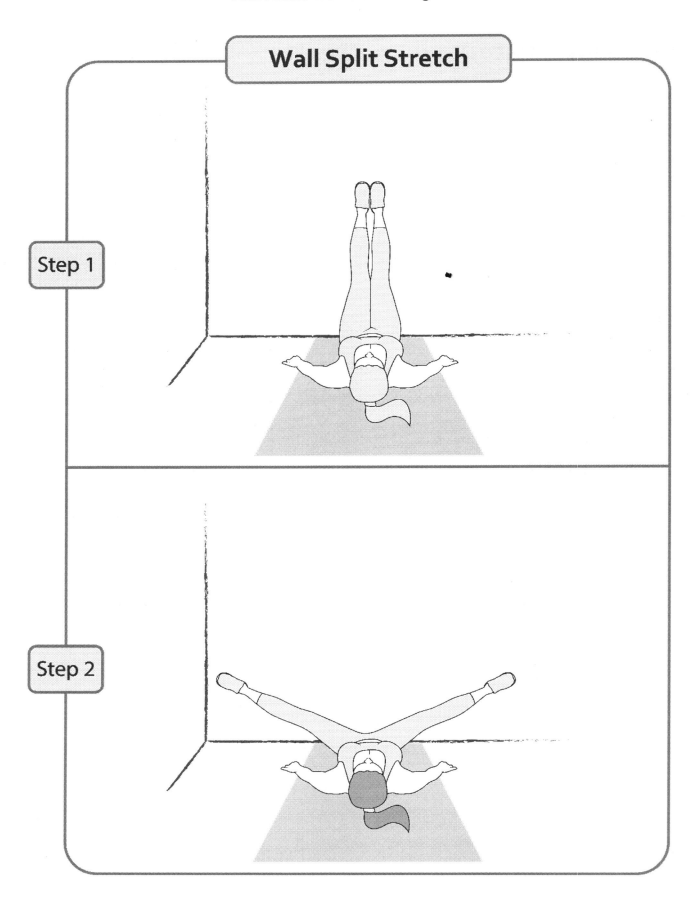

Step 2

Wall Split Stretch

Enhance Hamstring and Hip Flexibility

The Wall Split Stretch is designed to target hamstring and hip flexibility, helping you achieve a deeper split position. By using the wall for support, this exercise encourages proper alignment and allows you to focus on relaxing into the stretch.

Instructions:

1. Sit on the floor facing the wall, with your legs extended and your feet pressing against it.
2. Extend your legs as wide as you comfortably can, aiming to form a "V" shape.
3. Keep your core engaged to maintain proper posture.
4. Inhale deeply to lengthen your spine, and as you exhale, begin to lean your torso forward.
5. Walk your hands forward along the floor, aiming to reach your hands as far as possible.
6. Feel the stretch in your hamstrings and inner thighs.
7. Hold the stretch for the desired duration while continuing to breathe.
8. Inhale as you gently sit back up, using your hands for support.

Tips:

- *Keep your spine elongated and avoid rounding your back.*
- *Engage your core muscles to support your posture during the stretch.*
- *Breathe deeply and exhale to relax into the stretch.*
- *Aim for a gradual increase in the stretch as you exhale and lean forward.*
- *If you feel any pain, reduce the depth of the stretch and find a comfortable range.*
- *Focus on keeping both legs active and pressing against the wall for resistance.*
- *Consult a fitness professional if you have any concerns about your form or flexibility.*

The Wall Split Stretch is effective for enhancing hamstring and hip flexibility. As with any stretch, prioritize proper alignment and listen to your body's feedback.

Wall Chest Opener

Step 1

Step 2

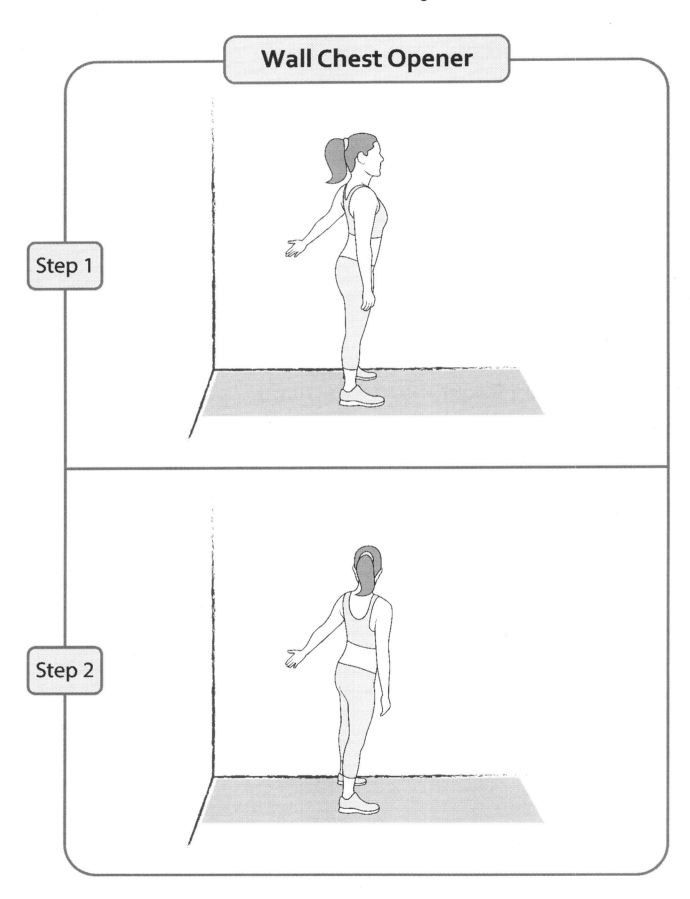

Wall Chest Opener

Improve Chest and Shoulder Mobility

The Wall Chest Opener focuses on improving chest and shoulder mobility while also stretching the front of the shoulders and chest muscles. Using the wall for support, this exercise helps counteract the effects of poor posture and encourages an open and balanced upper body.

Instructions:

1. Stand facing the wall and extend your arm to the side, palm against the wall at shoulder height.
2. Step slightly closer to the wall and rotate your body away from the arm that's extended.
3. Keep your arm extended and gently press your palm into the wall.
4. As you press your palm, begin to rotate your torso away from the arm, opening your chest.
5. Feel the stretch across the front of your shoulder and chest.
6. Hold the stretch for the desired duration while maintaining steady breathing.
7. Release the stretch and switch to the other arm, repeating the exercise.

Tips:

- *Keep your core engaged to support your spine and posture during the stretch.*
- *Avoid overarching your lower back; aim for a neutral spine.*
- *Breathe deeply and relax into the stretch as you exhale.*
- *Gently increase the stretch as you press your palm into the wall.*
- *Focus on maintaining a balanced posture throughout the exercise.*
- *If you experience discomfort, reduce the intensity of the stretch.*
- *Consult a fitness professional if you have any concerns about your form or mobility.*

The Wall Chest Opener is beneficial for improving chest and shoulder mobility, especially if you spend extended periods of time seated or working at a computer.

Wall Back Extension

Step 1

Step 2

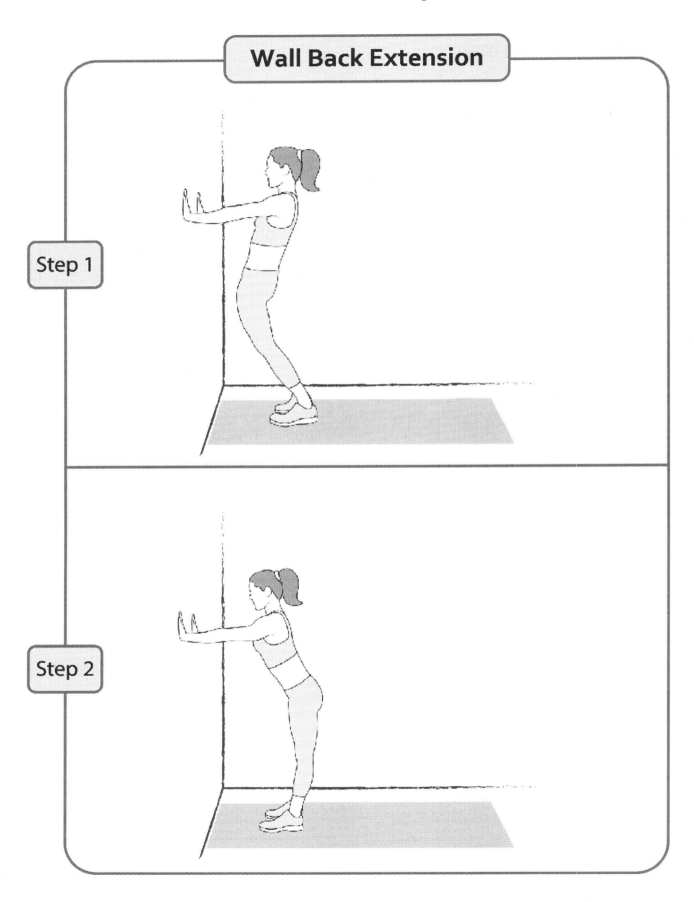

Wall Back Extension

Strengthen Back Muscles and Improve Posture

The Wall Back Extension is designed to strengthen the muscles along your spine and improve overall posture. By using the wall for support, you can focus on activating the muscles of your back and engaging your core while performing controlled extensions.

Instructions:

1. Stand facing the wall and place your hands against it at shoulder height.
2. Step back a short distance, creating a slight angle between your body and the wall.
3. Keep your feet hip-width apart and engage your core muscles.
4. Inhale as you lengthen your spine, and as you exhale, begin to lean your torso forward.
5. Keep your arms extended and your hands pressing into the wall.
6. Continue to lean forward until you feel a gentle stretch in your back.
7. Inhale as you return to an upright position, engaging your back muscles.
8. Exhale and perform a slight backward movement, arching your back while keeping your core engaged.

Tips:

- *Maintain a neutral spine and avoid excessive arching or rounding of your back.*
- *Engage your core muscles to support your posture during the exercise.*
- *Breathe deeply, exhaling as you lean forward and inhaling as you return to upright.*
- *Focus on a controlled and deliberate movement.*
- *Keep your shoulders relaxed and away from your ears.*
- *Gradually increase the depth of the forward lean as you feel more comfortable.*
- *Consult a fitness professional if you have any concerns about your form or back health.*

The Wall Back Extension is effective for strengthening the muscles of the back and promoting better posture. Prioritize proper form and listen to your body's feedback.

Wall Oblique Twist

Step 1

Step 2

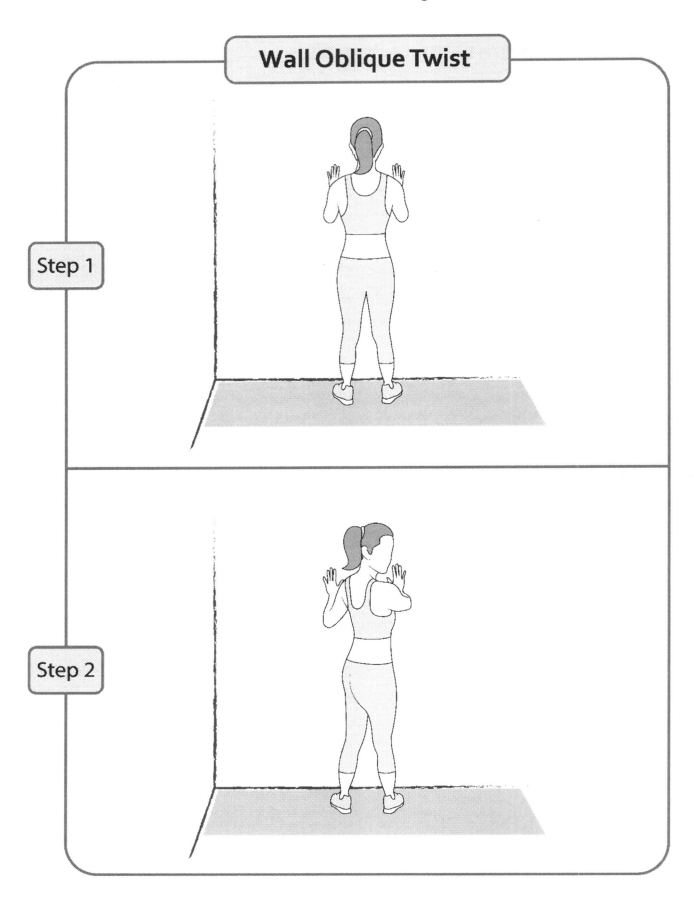

Wall Oblique Twist

Engage Oblique Muscles and Core

The Wall Oblique Twist targets the oblique muscles, which run along the sides of your abdomen. By using the wall for support, this exercise allows you to focus on controlled twisting movements that engage the obliques and contribute to improved core strength and stability.

Instructions:

1. Stand facing the wall, about arms' length away.
2. Extend your arms forward, parallel to the ground, and press your palms against the wall.
3. Position your feet hip-width apart and engage your core muscles.
4. Inhale deeply to prepare, and as you exhale, rotate your torso to one side.
5. Keep your hips facing forward and initiate the movement from your waist.
6. Inhale as you return to the center, and exhale as you rotate to the other side.
7. Continue alternating twists for the desired number of repetitions.

Tips:

- *Keep your core engaged throughout the exercise for stability.*
- *Focus on controlled twisting movements, avoiding jerky motions.*
- *Breathe naturally, exhaling as you rotate and inhaling as you return to the center.*
- *Maintain a neutral spine and avoid excessive twisting of the hips.*
- *Keep your arms extended and maintain gentle pressure against the wall.*
- *Gradually increase the range of motion as you feel more comfortable.*
- *Consult a fitness professional if you have any concerns about your form or any existing conditions.*

The Wall Oblique Twist is effective for engaging the oblique muscles and enhancing core strength.

Wall Calf Stretch

Step 1

Step 2

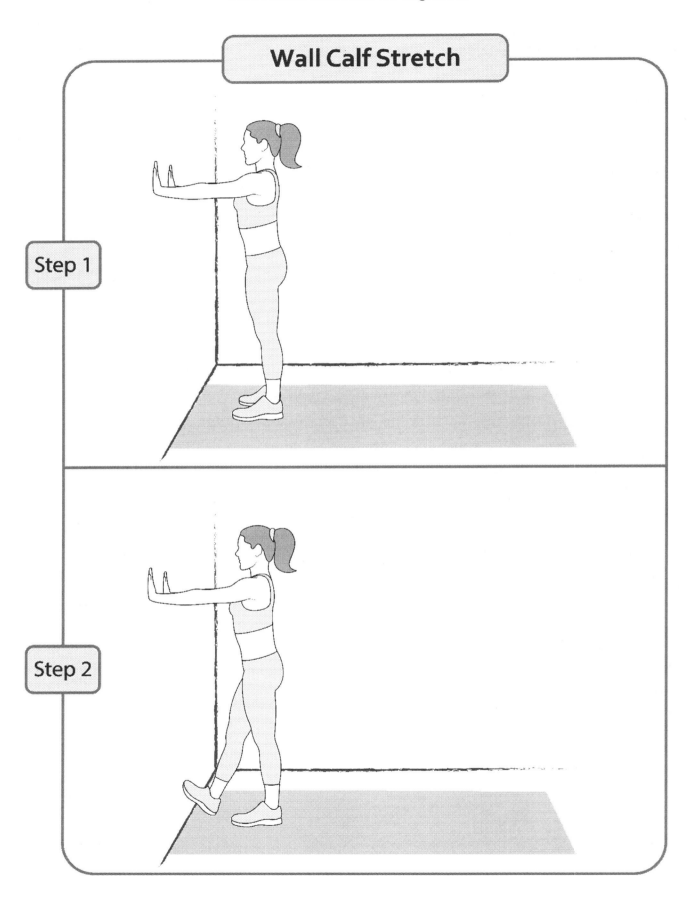

Wall Calf Stretch

Improve Lower Leg Flexibility

The Wall Calf Stretch focuses on improving flexibility in the calf muscles and the Achilles tendon. By using the wall for support, this stretch allows you to target the muscles at the back of the lower leg effectively.

Instructions:

1. Stand facing the wall, a comfortable distance away.
2. Place your hands against the wall at shoulder height for support.
3. Step one foot forward, keeping the other foot back with your heel on the ground.
4. Keep your back leg straight and your toes pointing forward.
5. Lean your hips and chest slightly toward the wall, feeling the stretch in your calf.
6. Hold the stretch for the desired duration while maintaining steady breathing.
7. Switch legs and repeat the stretch with the opposite leg.

Tips:

- *Keep your back heel on the ground throughout the stretch.*
- *Engage your core muscles to maintain proper posture.*
- *Breathe deeply and relax into the stretch as you exhale.*
- *Focus on feeling the stretch along the back of your calf.*
- *Gradually increase the depth of the stretch as you exhale and relax.*
- *Consult a fitness professional if you have any concerns about your form or flexibility.*

The Wall Calf Stretch is effective for improving flexibility in the calf muscles and promoting better lower leg mobility. Practice with proper form and listen to your body's feedback during the stretch.

Wall Split Squat

Step 1

Step 2

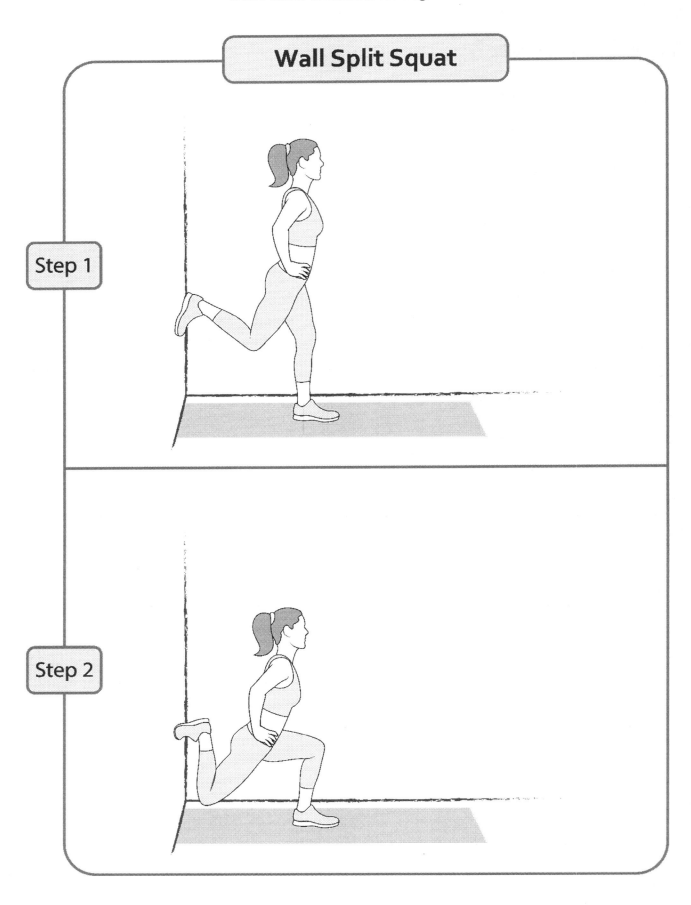

Wall Split Squat

Strengthen Legs and Improve Balance

The Wall Split Squat is designed to strengthen the legs, particularly the quadriceps and glutes, while also improving balance and stability. By using the wall for support, this exercise allows you to focus on proper form and controlled movements.

Instructions:

1. Stand facing away from the wall, a comfortable distance away.
2. Extend one leg behind you and rest the top of your foot against the wall.
3. Position your front leg with a bent knee, creating a lunge-like stance.
4. Engage your core muscles for stability.
5. Inhale as you lower your back knee toward the ground, creating a lunge position.
6. Exhale as you push through your front heel to return to the starting position.
7. Perform the desired number of repetitions on one leg before switching sides.

Tips:

- *Keep your front knee aligned with your ankle and avoid letting it go past your toes.*
- *Engage your core muscles throughout the exercise for balance and stability.*
- *Focus on controlled movements, lowering and lifting with control.*
- *Breathe naturally during the exercise.*
- *Keep your shoulders relaxed and away from your ears.*
- *If you need extra support, lightly rest your fingertips against the wall.*
- *Gradually increase the depth of the squat as your strength and flexibility improve.*

The Wall Split Squat is effective for strengthening the legs and enhancing lower body stability.

Wall Arabesque

Step 1

Step 2

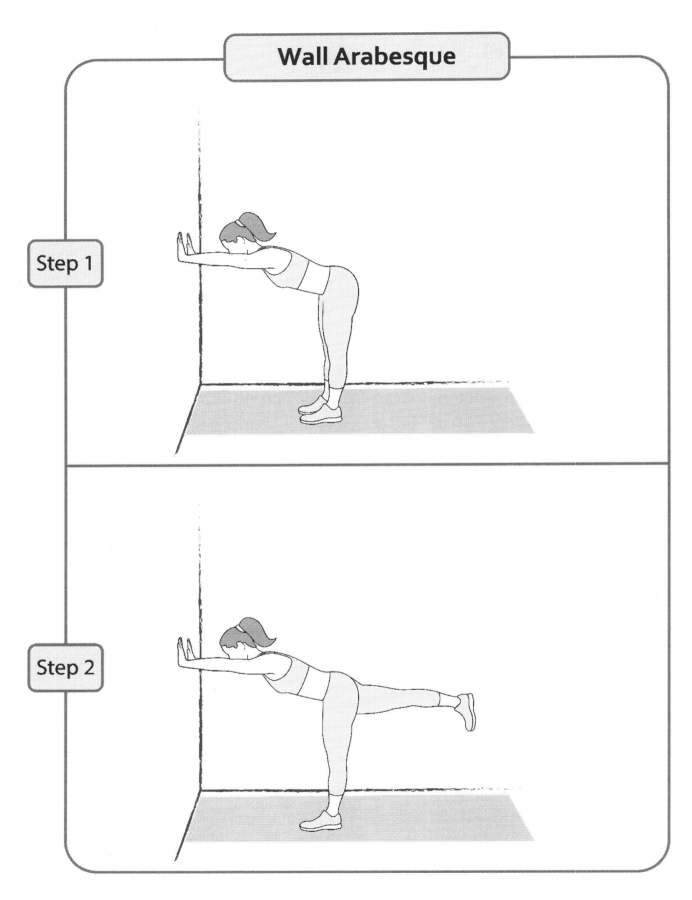

Wall Arabesque

Target Glutes and Improve Leg Extension

The Wall Arabesque focuses on strengthening the glutes and improving leg extension. By using the wall for support, you can maintain proper alignment and concentrate on controlled movements that engage the muscles of the lower body.

Instructions:

1. Stand facing the wall, a short distance away, with your hands lightly resting on the wall for support.
2. Shift your weight to one leg and extend the opposite leg behind you.
3. Keep your extended leg straight and your toes pointed.
4. Engage your core muscles for stability.
5. Inhale as you lift your back leg upward, squeezing your glutes.
6. Exhale as you lower your leg back down, maintaining control.
7. Perform the desired number of repetitions on one leg before switching sides.

Tips:

- *Keep your hips level and avoid tilting to one side.*
- *Engage your core muscles throughout the exercise for stability.*
- *Focus on lifting your leg with control, emphasizing the contraction of your glutes.*
- *Breathe naturally during the exercise.*
- *Keep your shoulders relaxed and maintain proper posture.*
- *Use the wall for balance as needed, but aim to engage your leg muscles for control.*
- *Gradually increase the height of your leg lift as your strength improves.*

The Wall Arabesque is effective for engaging the glutes and improving leg extension.

Handstand against a wall

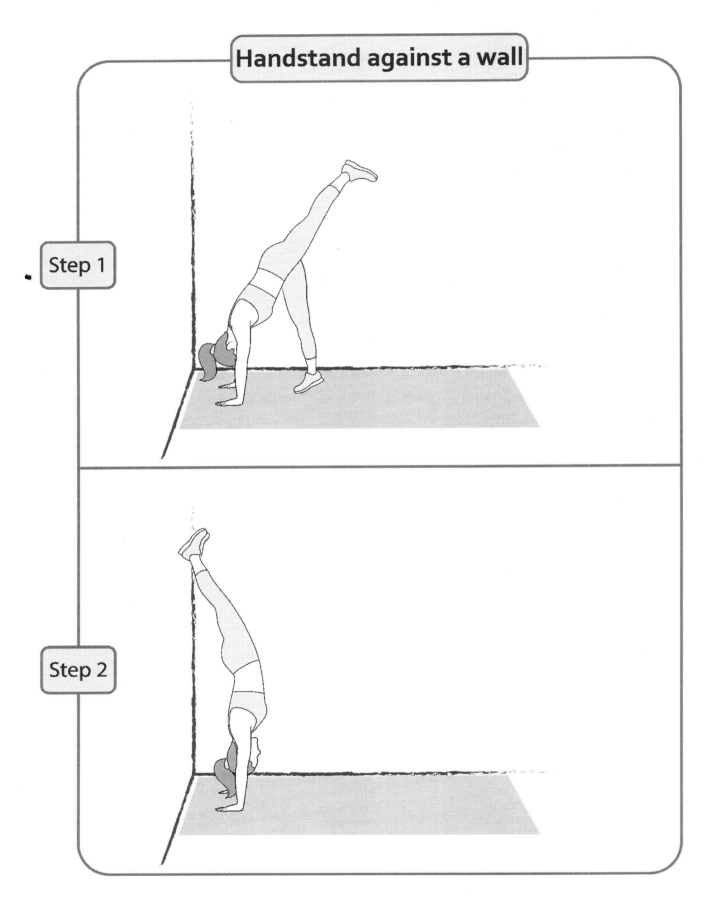

Step 1

Step 2

Handstand Against the Wall

Improving blood circulation and enriching the brain with oxygen

The Handstand Against the Wall is a challenging but rewarding exercise that builds strength, balance, and body awareness. Performing this exercise safely is essential. A handstand against a wall involves balancing on your hands while your body is inverted, with your feet resting on the wall for support.

Instructions:

1. Start in a kneeling position facing the wall, about a foot away from it.
2. Place your hands on the floor shoulder-width apart, fingers spread wide, and your palms flat.
3. Ensure your wrists are directly under your shoulders.
4. Shift your weight forward onto your hands.
5. Begin to kick one leg up gently, aiming to get your heel to touch the wall.
6. As your first leg reaches the wall, use the momentum to kick your second leg up.
7. Both feet should eventually rest against the wall, and your body should be inverted in a straight line.
8. In the handstand position, focus on keeping your body in a straight line from your wrists to your ankles.
9. Engage your core muscles to maintain stability.
10. Keep your head in a neutral position, looking between your hands.
11. Once in the handstand position, hold it for as long as you can comfortably.
12. When you're ready to come down, tuck your knees into your chest.
13. Gently and with control, lower one foot to the floor at a time.

Tips:

- *It's advisable to have a spotter or practice with someone experienced, especially when starting.*
- *Keep your movements controlled and avoid kicking up with excessive force.*
- *If you feel any strain or discomfort, come down immediately.*
- *Consistency is key in mastering handstands; progress may be slow but will come with practice.*

Performing a handstand against a wall requires patience and perseverance. Always prioritize safety and proper form, and consider seeking guidance from a certified gymnastics or yoga instructor if you're new to handstands.

30-Day Wall Pilates Challenge

Welcome to the 30-Day Wall Pilates Challenge! This challenge is designed to help you build strength, flexibility, and body awareness using a variety of Wall Pilates exercises. Over the next 30 days, you'll progressively work through a range of movements, targeting different muscle groups and gradually increasing the intensity. Are you ready to commit to transforming your body and mind? Let's get started!

Challenge Guidelines:

- Perform the designated exercises for each day.
- Aim for proper form and controlled movements in every exercise.
- Adjust the number of sets and repetitions to match your fitness level.
- Always warm up before you start and cool down/stretch after each session.
- Listen to your body; if an exercise causes discomfort or pain, modify or skip it.
- Stay hydrated and maintain a balanced diet to support your challenge.

Day 1-5: Core Foundation

1. Wall Roll Down: 3 sets of 6 repetitions
2. Wall Pike: Hold for 10 seconds, rest for 10 seconds; repeat 3 times
3. Wall Push-Ups: 2 sets of 10 repetitions
4. Wall Bridge: 2 sets of 8 repetitions
5. Wall Plank: Hold for 15 seconds, rest for 10 seconds; repeat 3 times

Day 6-10: Upper Body Empowerment

6. Wall Triceps Dips: 2 sets of 8 repetitions
7. Wall Pike Roll Down: 3 sets of 6 repetitions
8. Wall Arm Circles: 2 sets of 10 repetitions
9. Wall Push-Up with Leg Lift: 2 sets of 8 repetitions
10. Wall Teaser: 2 sets of 6 repetitions

Day 11-15: Lower Body Strength

11. Wall Squats: 3 sets of 12 repetitions
12. Wall Single Leg Stretch: 2 sets of 8 repetitions on each leg
13. Wall Lunge Stretch: Hold for 20 seconds on each leg; repeat 2 times

14. Wall Side Leg Lifts: 2 sets of 8 repetitions on each leg

15. Wall Split Squat: 2 sets of 8 repetitions on each leg

Day 16-20: Total Body Sculpt

16. Wall Pike: Hold for 12 seconds, rest for 8 seconds; repeat 4 times

17. Wall Scissor: 2 sets of 10 repetitions on each leg

18. Wall Arabesque: 2 sets of 10 repetitions on each leg

19. Wall Side Plank: Hold for 15 seconds on each side; repeat 2 times

20. Wall Corkscrew: 2 sets of 8 repetitions

Day 21-25: Core Mastery

21. Wall Pike Roll Down: 3 sets of 6 repetitions

22. Wall Torso Rotation: 2 sets of 10 repetitions on each side

23. Wall Oblique Twist: 2 sets of 12 repetitions on each side

24. Wall Roll Up: 2 sets of 8 repetitions

25. Wall Pike: Hold for 15 seconds, rest for 10 seconds; repeat 4 times

Day 26-30: Flexibility and Relaxation

26. Wall Mermaid Stretch: Hold for 20 seconds on each side; repeat 2 times

27. Wall Split Stretch: Hold for 25 seconds on each leg; repeat 2 times

28. Wall Chest Opener: Hold for 20 seconds; repeat 2 times

29. Wall Back Extension: 2 sets of 8 repetitions

30. Wall Calf Stretch: Hold for 30 seconds on each leg; repeat 2 times

Congratulations on Completing the Challenge!

As you wrap up the 30-Day Wall Pilates Challenge, take a moment to celebrate your accomplishments. You've dedicated yourself to enhancing your strength, flexibility, and overall well-being. This challenge is just the beginning of your journey toward a healthier and more mindful lifestyle. Feel free to continue practicing these exercises and exploring new variations to maintain your progress. Your commitment to this challenge demonstrates your dedication to self-care and personal growth. Keep moving, keep breathing, and enjoy the transformative effects of Wall Pilates in your life!

Cooling Down and Stretching

As your Wall Pilates workouts come to an end, it's important to allow your body to gradually transition from exercise mode to a state of relaxation. This chapter focuses on the essential cooling down and stretching routine that follows your Wall Pilates sessions. Cooling down and stretching contribute to reducing muscle tension, promoting flexibility, and aiding in recovery. By incorporating these practices, you'll ensure a well-rounded and holistic experience.

The Importance of Cooling Down:

A proper cool-down is like a graceful conclusion to your workout, allowing your body to gradually return to its resting state. Cooling down has numerous benefits:

- **Reduced Muscle Stiffness:** It helps prevent the buildup of lactic acid, which can lead to muscle stiffness and soreness.

- **Promotion of Blood Flow:** Gentle movement during the cool-down promotes blood flow, aiding in the removal of waste products from muscles.

- **Transition to Resting State:** Cooling down prepares your body for rest and recovery, preventing abrupt changes that can strain your cardiovascular system.

Cooling Down Routine:

1. **March in Place:** March gently in place for about 2 minutes. This low-impact movement helps keep blood flowing while gradually decreasing your heart rate.

2. **Gentle Movement:** Perform easy, fluid movements such as shoulder rolls, wrist circles, and hip swings. This promotes joint mobility and prevents stiffness.

3. **Deep Breathing:** Spend a few minutes focusing on deep, diaphragmatic breathing. Inhale deeply through your nose, expand your belly, and exhale fully through your mouth.

The Importance of Stretching:

Stretching is an integral part of cooling down. It helps maintain and improve flexibility, enhances joint range of motion, and relaxes your muscles.

Stretching Routine:

1. **Wall Calf Stretch:** Stand facing the wall. Step one foot back and press the heel into the ground. Feel the stretch in your calf. Hold for 20-30 seconds per leg.

2. **Wall Hamstring Stretch:** Sit on the floor with one leg extended up the wall. Flex your foot and gently reach towards your extended foot. Hold for 20-30 seconds per leg.

3. **Wall Quadriceps Stretch:** Stand facing the wall. Bend one knee and grab your ankle behind you. Gently pull your heel towards your glutes, feeling the stretch in your quadriceps. Hold for 20-30 seconds per leg.

4. **Wall Chest Opener Stretch:** Stand facing the wall. Place one hand on the wall at shoulder height. Rotate your torso away from the wall, feeling the stretch across your chest and shoulders. Hold for 20-30 seconds per side.

5. **Wall Child's Pose:** Kneel facing the wall and extend your arms forward, resting your forehead on the wall. Feel the stretch in your spine and shoulders. Hold for 30 seconds.

Wrap-Up:

By dedicating a few minutes to cooling down and stretching after your Wall Pilates workouts, you're prioritizing your body's recovery and well-being. The cool-down routine gradually eases your body out of exercise mode, while the stretching routine enhances flexibility and relaxation. These practices not only contribute to your physical progress but also promote a sense of mindfulness and self-care. As you make cooling down and stretching a regular part of your Wall Pilates routine, you'll reap the rewards of enhanced mobility, reduced muscle tension, and a more balanced and harmonious body.

Incorporating Wall Pilates into Your Routine

In this chapter, you'll learn how to seamlessly integrate Wall Pilates into your daily life. As you've discovered the numerous benefits of Wall Pilates, you'll find that it's a versatile practice that can be adapted to your schedule, preferences, and fitness goals. Whether you're looking to make it a consistent part of your routine or mix it with other forms of exercise, this chapter will guide you in maximizing the impact of Wall Pilates on your overall well-being.

Finding the Right Frequency:

The frequency of your Wall Pilates practice depends on your fitness level, goals, and availability. Here are some guidelines to consider:

- **Beginners:** Start with 2-3 sessions per week to allow your body to adapt and recover.
- **Intermediate:** Aim for 3-4 sessions per week to continue building strength and flexibility.
- **Advanced:** 4-5 sessions per week can provide optimal results while allowing time for recovery.

Combining Wall Pilates with Other Forms of Exercise:

Wall Pilates can be a fantastic standalone practice or a complementary addition to your existing fitness routine. Here are some ideas for incorporating Wall Pilates into your overall wellness plan:

- **Cardiovascular Exercise:** Pair it with cardiovascular activities like walking, jogging, or cycling to create a balanced workout routine.
- **Strength Training:** Use Wall Pilates to enhance your core strength and flexibility, which can support your weightlifting or resistance training efforts.
- **Yoga and Meditation:** Combine it with yoga and meditation to create a holistic approach that addresses both physical and mental well-being.
- **Rest and Recovery:** On rest days, engage in gentle Wall Pilates exercises to promote blood flow and prevent stiffness.

Customizing Your Wall Pilates Routine:

Feel free to modify and tailor your routine to suit your individual preferences and needs:

- **Duration:** Adjust the length of your sessions based on your schedule and energy levels.
- **Focus:** Emphasize specific muscle groups or goals in your routine. For example, you can dedicate a session to core work or flexibility.

- **Variety:** Experiment with different exercises to keep your routine engaging and challenging.

Mindfulness and Progress:

Remember that consistency is key in any fitness journey. As you incorporate Wall Pilates into your routine, focus on the quality of your practice rather than rushing through the exercises. Mindful movement enhances your mind-body connection and ensures proper form.

Conclusion: Your Wall Pilates Lifestyle

Incorporating Wall Pilates into your routine is a commitment to your well-being. Whether you choose to practice it daily or a few times a week, each session contributes to your overall health and fitness. By combining Wall Pilates with other forms of exercise and embracing the versatility it offers, you'll embark on a journey of self-discovery and self-care.

As you move forward, adapt your routine to your changing needs and celebrate your progress. Remember that Wall Pilates is not just about physical transformation; it's about cultivating a balanced and harmonious lifestyle that supports your body, mind, and spirit. With dedication, patience, and the guidance you've acquired throughout this book, you're well on your way to experiencing the lasting benefits of Wall Pilates in your life.

The Pilates Practitioner's Guide to Optimal Nutrition

Pilates is not just a workout; it's a holistic approach to physical fitness and well-being. As you engage in this discipline to strengthen your core, improve flexibility, and enhance your overall body awareness, it's crucial to fuel your body properly. Nutrition plays a vital role in maximizing the benefits of Pilates and promoting your overall health. In this guide, we'll explore the key principles of nutrition for Pilates practitioners.

Stay Hydrated

Before diving into the intricacies of dietary choices, let's start with the foundation of good nutrition - hydration. Staying well-hydrated is essential for optimal Pilates performance. Dehydration can lead to muscle cramps, decreased flexibility, and reduced endurance. Aim to drink water throughout the day, and hydrate before, during, and after your Pilates sessions.

Balance Your Macronutrients

To maintain energy levels during your Pilates sessions and throughout the day, it's essential to consume a balanced mix of macronutrients:

- **Carbohydrates:** These are your body's primary energy source. Opt for complex carbohydrates like whole grains, fruits, and vegetables, which provide sustained energy.

- **Proteins:** Protein is crucial for muscle repair and growth. Include lean sources such as poultry, fish, tofu, beans, and nuts in your diet.

- **Fats:** Healthy fats are essential for overall health. Incorporate sources like avocados, olive oil, nuts, and fatty fish for improved joint flexibility and brain function.

Prioritize Pre-Workout Nutrition

To get the most out of your Pilates sessions, fuel up with a balanced meal or snack 1-2 hours before your workout. A combination of carbohydrates and protein can provide sustained energy. For example, try a banana with almond butter or Greek yogurt with berries.

Post-Workout Recovery

After your Pilates session, it's crucial to support your body's recovery process. Consume a meal or snack that includes protein and carbohydrates within 2 hours of your workout. This aids in muscle repair and replenishes glycogen stores. A turkey and vegetable wrap or a smoothie with protein powder and spinach are great options.

Listen to Your Body

Pilates enhances body awareness, and this extends to your dietary choices. Pay attention to your body's signals of hunger and fullness. Eating mindfully can help you avoid overeating and make more conscious choices about what you eat.

Avoid Heavy Meals Before Pilates

While it's essential to fuel your body, avoid consuming heavy or large meals immediately before your Pilates session. This can lead to discomfort and reduced flexibility during your workout. Instead, opt for a light snack if you're hungry.

Embrace Whole Foods

Whole foods like fruits, vegetables, whole grains, and lean proteins should form the foundation of your diet. They provide essential nutrients, fiber, and antioxidants that support overall health and recovery.

Control Your Portions

Paying attention to portion sizes can help you maintain a healthy weight and prevent discomfort during Pilates. Use visual cues like your hand or a measuring cup to gauge appropriate portion sizes.

Consider Supplementation

While it's best to obtain nutrients from whole foods, some Pilates practitioners may benefit from supplements. Consult with a healthcare provider or registered dietitian to determine if you have specific nutritional needs.

Be Mindful of Special Diets

If you have dietary restrictions or follow a special diet (e.g., vegetarian, vegan, gluten-free), it's essential to plan your meals carefully to ensure you're meeting your nutritional needs. Consulting with a dietitian can be particularly helpful in these cases.

Limit Processed Foods

Processed foods, high in added sugars, unhealthy fats, and sodium, can contribute to inflammation and discomfort. Minimize your intake of these items and focus on whole, unprocessed foods.

Stay Consistent

Consistency is key to reaping the long-term benefits of Pilates and good nutrition. Develop healthy eating habits that align with your Pilates practice and your overall health goals.

In conclusion, Pilates and nutrition go hand in hand. By fueling your body with the right nutrients and staying hydrated, you can optimize your Pilates sessions, support muscle recovery, and promote overall well-being. Remember that nutrition is a personal journey, and what works best for one person may differ for another. Listen to your body, stay mindful of your dietary choices, and consult with a healthcare provider or registered dietitian if you have specific dietary concerns or goals. With a balanced approach to nutrition, you can enhance your Pilates practice and enjoy improved vitality and health.

★ ★ ★ BONUS CHAPTER ★ ★ ★

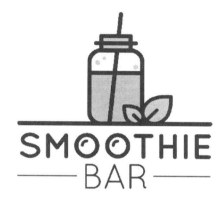

Only the best smoothie recipes

As a bonus, we have added a chapter with recipes for healthy smoothies that will help your body replenish its stores of nutrients and vitamins. Smoothies also help you lose weight and normalize your metabolism. This chapter contains only the best and most effective recipes, which together with exercises will help to improve your figure, health, and well-being. Enjoy the variety of flavors!

Berry Bliss Smoothie

Preparation time: 5 minutes

Servings: 2

Ingredients:
- 1 cup fresh or frozen mixed berries (strawberries, blueberries, raspberries, and blackberries)
- 1 small banana, peeled and sliced
- 1 cup baby spinach or kale
- 1/2 cup Greek yogurt or dairy-free yogurt alternative
- 1/2 cup unsweetened almond milk or any non-dairy milk of your choice
- 1 tablespoon chia seeds or ground flaxseeds
- 1 tablespoon honey or pure maple syrup (optional)
- 1/2 teaspoon ground turmeric
- 1/4 teaspoon ground cinnamon
- A pinch of ground black pepper
- A few ice cubes (optional)

Instructions:
1. In a blender, combine the mixed berries, banana, baby spinach or kale, yogurt, almond milk or non-dairy milk, chia seeds or ground flaxseeds, honey or maple syrup (if using), ground turmeric, ground cinnamon, and ground black pepper.
2. Blend on high speed until the mixture is smooth, creamy, and well combined. Add ice cubes if you prefer a colder and thicker texture.
3. Taste the smoothie and adjust the sweetness or seasoning as needed. If the smoothie is too thick, add a little more almond milk or non-dairy milk to achieve the desired consistency.
4. Pour the smoothie into two glasses and serve immediately. Enjoy this refreshing and nutritious smoothie for breakfast or as a snack.

Nutrients per serving:
- Calories: ~185 kcal
- Protein: ~7 g
- Fat: ~4 g
- Carbohydrates: ~33 g
- Fiber: ~7 g

Orange Sunshine Smoothie

Preparation time: 5 minutes
Servings: 2

Ingredients:
- 1 large orange, peeled and segmented
- 1 small carrot, peeled and chopped
- 1 small banana, peeled and sliced
- 1/2 cup frozen or fresh pineapple chunks
- 1/2 cup Greek yogurt or dairy-free yogurt alternative
- 1 cup unsweetened almond milk or any non-dairy milk of your choice
- 1 tablespoon chia seeds or ground flaxseeds
- 1/2 teaspoon ground turmeric
- 1/4 teaspoon ground cinnamon
- A pinch of ground black pepper
- A few ice cubes (optional)

Instructions:
1. In a blender, combine the orange segments, chopped carrot, banana, pineapple chunks, yogurt, almond milk or non-dairy milk, chia seeds or ground flaxseeds, ground turmeric, ground cinnamon, and ground black pepper.
2. Blend on high speed until the mixture is smooth, creamy, and well combined. Add ice cubes if you prefer a colder and thicker texture.
3. Taste the smoothie and adjust the seasoning as needed. If the smoothie is too thick, add a little more almond milk or non-dairy milk to achieve the desired consistency.
4. Pour the smoothie into two glasses and serve immediately. Enjoy this refreshing and nutritious smoothie for breakfast or as a snack.

Nutrients per serving:
- Calories: ~195 kcal
- Protein: ~7 g
- Fat: ~4 g
- Carbohydrates: ~35 g
- Fiber: ~6 g

Blueberry Avocado Smoothie

Preparation time: 5 minutes
Servings: 2

Ingredients:
- 1 cup fresh or frozen blueberries
- 1/2 ripe avocado, peeled and pitted
- 1 small banana, peeled and sliced
- 1 cup baby spinach or kale
- 1 tablespoon chia seeds or ground flaxseeds
- 1 cup unsweetened almond milk or any non-dairy milk of your choice
- 1 tablespoon honey or pure maple syrup (optional)
- 1/2 teaspoon ground turmeric
- 1/4 teaspoon ground cinnamon
- A pinch of ground black pepper
- A few ice cubes (optional)

Instructions:
1. In a blender, combine the blueberries, avocado, banana, baby spinach or kale, chia seeds or ground flaxseeds, almond milk or non-dairy milk, honey or maple syrup (if using), ground turmeric, ground cinnamon, and ground black pepper.
2. Blend on high speed until the mixture is smooth, creamy, and well combined. Add ice cubes if you prefer a colder and thicker texture.
3. Taste the smoothie and adjust the sweetness or seasoning as needed. If the smoothie is too thick, add a little more almond milk or non-dairy milk to achieve the desired consistency.
4. Pour the smoothie into two glasses and serve immediately. Enjoy this refreshing and nutritious smoothie for breakfast or as a snack.

Nutrients per serving:
- Calories: ~240 kcal
- Protein: ~5 g
- Fat: ~12 g
- Carbohydrates: ~31 g
- Fiber: ~9 g

Cherry Almond Smoothie

Preparation time: 5 minutes
Servings: 2

Ingredients:
- 1 cup fresh or frozen pitted cherries
- 1 small banana, peeled and sliced
- 1/4 cup raw almonds or 2 tablespoons almond butter
- 1 cup baby spinach or kale
- 1 tablespoon chia seeds or ground flaxseeds
- 1 cup unsweetened almond milk or any non-dairy milk of your choice
- 1 tablespoon honey or pure maple syrup (optional)
- 1/2 teaspoon ground turmeric
- 1/4 teaspoon ground cinnamon
- A pinch of ground black pepper
- A few ice cubes (optional)

Instructions:
1. In a blender, combine the cherries, banana, almonds or almond butter, baby spinach or kale, chia seeds or ground flaxseeds, almond milk or non-dairy milk, honey or maple syrup (if using), ground turmeric, ground cinnamon, and ground black pepper.
2. Blend on high speed until the mixture is smooth, creamy, and well combined. Add ice cubes if you prefer a colder and thicker texture.
3. Taste the smoothie and adjust the sweetness or seasoning as needed. If the smoothie is too thick, add a little more almond milk or non-dairy milk to achieve the desired consistency.
4. Pour the smoothie into two glasses and serve immediately. Enjoy this refreshing and nutritious smoothie for breakfast or as a snack.

Nutrients per serving:
- Calories: ~250 kcal
- Protein: ~7 g
- Fat: ~12 g
- Carbohydrates: ~32 g
- Fiber: ~7 g

Apple Cinnamon Smoothie

Preparation time: 5 minutes
Servings: 2

Ingredients:
- 1 medium apple, cored and chopped
- 1 small banana, peeled and sliced
- 1/2 cup Greek yogurt or dairy-free yogurt alternative
- 1 cup unsweetened almond milk or any non-dairy milk of your choice
- 1 tablespoon chia seeds or ground flaxseeds
- 1/2 teaspoon ground cinnamon
- 1/4 teaspoon ground ginger
- A pinch of ground nutmeg
- A few ice cubes (optional)

Instructions:
1. In a blender, combine the chopped apple, banana, yogurt, almond milk or non-dairy milk, chia seeds or ground flaxseeds, ground cinnamon, ground ginger, and ground nutmeg.
2. Blend on high speed until the mixture is smooth, creamy, and well combined. Add ice cubes if you prefer a colder and thicker texture.
3. Taste the smoothie and adjust the seasoning as needed. If the smoothie is too thick, add a little more almond milk or non-dairy milk to achieve the desired consistency.
4. Pour the smoothie into two glasses and serve immediately. Enjoy this refreshing and nutritious smoothie for breakfast or as a snack.

Nutrients per serving:
- Calories: ~190 kcal
- Protein: ~8 g
- Fat: ~5 g
- Carbohydrates: ~32 g
- Fiber: ~6 g

Berry Bliss Smoothie

Preparation time: 5 minutes
Servings: 2

Ingredients:
- 1 cup mixed fresh or frozen berries (such as strawberries, raspberries, blueberries, and blackberries)
- 1 small banana, peeled and sliced
- 1 cup baby spinach or kale
- 1 tablespoon chia seeds or ground flaxseeds
- 1 cup unsweetened almond milk or any non-dairy milk of your choice
- 1 tablespoon honey or pure maple syrup (optional)
- 1/2 teaspoon ground turmeric
- A pinch of ground black pepper
- A few ice cubes (optional)

Instructions:
1. In a blender, combine the mixed berries, banana, baby spinach or kale, chia seeds or ground flaxseeds, almond milk or non-dairy milk, honey or maple syrup (if using), ground turmeric, and ground black pepper.

2. Blend on high speed until the mixture is smooth, creamy, and well combined. Add ice cubes if you prefer a colder and thicker texture.

3. Taste the smoothie and adjust the sweetness or seasoning as needed. If the smoothie is too thick, add a little more almond milk or non-dairy milk to achieve the desired consistency.

4. Pour the smoothie into two glasses and serve immediately. Enjoy this refreshing and nutritious smoothie for breakfast or as a snack.

Nutrients per serving:
- Calories: ~160 kcal
- Protein: ~4 g
- Fat: ~4 g
- Carbohydrates: ~30 g
- Fiber: ~6 g

Tropical Green Smoothie

Preparation time: 5 minutes
Servings: 2

Ingredients:
- 1 cup fresh or frozen pineapple chunks
- 1/2 cup fresh or frozen mango chunks
- 1 small banana, peeled and sliced
- 1 cup baby spinach or kale
- 1 tablespoon chia seeds or ground flaxseeds
- 1 cup unsweetened coconut milk or any non-dairy milk of your choice
- 1 tablespoon honey or pure maple syrup (optional)
- 1/2 teaspoon ground turmeric
- A pinch of ground black pepper
- A few ice cubes (optional)

Instructions:
1. In a blender, combine the pineapple chunks, mango chunks, banana, baby spinach or kale, chia seeds or ground flaxseeds, coconut milk or non-dairy milk, honey or maple syrup (if using), ground turmeric, and ground black pepper.
2. Blend on high speed until the mixture is smooth, creamy, and well combined. Add ice cubes if you prefer a colder and thicker texture.
3. Taste the smoothie and adjust the sweetness or seasoning as needed. If the smoothie is too thick, add a little more coconut milk or non-dairy milk to achieve the desired consistency.
4. Pour the smoothie into two glasses and serve immediately. Enjoy this refreshing and nutritious smoothie for breakfast or as a snack.

Nutrients per serving:
- Calories: ~230 kcal
- Protein: ~4 g
- Fat: ~9 g
- Carbohydrates: ~36 g
- Fiber: ~5 g

Orange Carrot Ginger Smoothie

Preparation time: 5 minutes
Servings: 2

Ingredients:
- 1 medium orange, peeled and segmented
- 1 medium carrot, peeled and chopped
- 1 small banana, peeled and sliced
- 1/2 inch piece of fresh ginger, peeled and grated
- 1 tablespoon chia seeds or ground flaxseeds
- 1 cup unsweetened almond milk or any non-dairy milk of your choice
- 1 tablespoon honey or pure maple syrup (optional)
- 1/2 teaspoon ground turmeric
- A pinch of ground black pepper
- A few ice cubes (optional)

Instructions:
1. In a blender, combine the orange segments, chopped carrot, banana, grated ginger, chia seeds or ground flaxseeds, almond milk or non-dairy milk, honey or maple syrup (if using), ground turmeric, and ground black pepper.
2. Blend on high speed until the mixture is smooth, creamy, and well combined. Add ice cubes if you prefer a colder and thicker texture.
3. Taste the smoothie and adjust the sweetness or seasoning as needed. If the smoothie is too thick, add a little more almond milk or non-dairy milk to achieve the desired consistency.
4. Pour the smoothie into two glasses and serve immediately. Enjoy this refreshing and nutritious smoothie for breakfast or as a snack.

Nutrients per serving:
- Calories: ~180 kcal
- Protein: ~4 g
- Fat: ~4 g
- Carbohydrates: ~34 g
- Fiber: ~6 g

Blueberry Avocado Smoothie

Preparation time: 5 minutes
Servings: 2

Ingredients:
- 1 cup fresh or frozen blueberries
- 1/2 medium avocado, peeled and pitted
- 1 small banana, peeled and sliced
- 1 cup baby spinach or kale
- 1 tablespoon chia seeds or ground flaxseeds
- 1 cup unsweetened almond milk or any non-dairy milk of your choice
- 1 tablespoon honey or pure maple syrup (optional)
- 1/2 teaspoon ground turmeric
- A pinch of ground black pepper
- A few ice cubes (optional)

Instructions:
1. In a blender, combine the blueberries, avocado, banana, baby spinach or kale, chia seeds or ground flaxseeds, almond milk or non-dairy milk, honey or maple syrup (if using), ground turmeric, and ground black pepper.
2. Blend on high speed until the mixture is smooth, creamy, and well combined. Add ice cubes if you prefer a colder and thicker texture.
3. Taste the smoothie and adjust the sweetness or seasoning as needed. If the smoothie is too thick, add a little more almond milk or non-dairy milk to achieve the desired consistency.
4. Pour the smoothie into two glasses and serve immediately. Enjoy this refreshing and nutritious smoothie for breakfast or as a snack.

Nutrients per serving:
- Calories: ~220 kcal
- Protein: ~5 g
- Fat: ~10 g
- Carbohydrates: ~30 g
- Fiber: ~8 g

Peach Ginger Smoothie

Preparation time: 5 minutes
Servings: 2

Ingredients:
- 1 cup fresh or frozen peach slices
- 1 small banana, peeled and sliced
- 1/2 inch piece of fresh ginger, peeled and grated
- 1 cup baby spinach or kale
- 1 tablespoon chia seeds or ground flaxseeds
- 1 cup unsweetened almond milk or any non-dairy milk of your choice
- 1 tablespoon honey or pure maple syrup (optional)
- 1/2 teaspoon ground turmeric
- A pinch of ground black pepper
- A few ice cubes (optional)

Instructions:
1. In a blender, combine the peach slices, banana, grated ginger, baby spinach or kale, chia seeds or ground flaxseeds, almond milk or non-dairy milk, honey or maple syrup (if using), ground turmeric, and ground black pepper.
2. Blend on high speed until the mixture is smooth, creamy, and well combined. Add ice cubes if you prefer a colder and thicker texture.
3. Taste the smoothie and adjust the sweetness or seasoning as needed. If the smoothie is too thick, add a little more almond milk or non-dairy milk to achieve the desired consistency.
4. Pour the smoothie into two glasses and serve immediately. Enjoy this refreshing and nutritious smoothie for breakfast or as a snack.

Nutrients per serving:
- Calories: ~170 kcal
- Protein: ~4 g
- Fat: ~4 g
- Carbohydrates: ~32 g
- Fiber: ~6 g

Kiwi Cucumber Smoothie

Preparation time: 5 minutes
Servings: 2

Ingredients:
- 2 kiwifruit, peeled and chopped
- 1/2 medium cucumber, peeled and chopped
- 1 small banana, peeled and sliced
- 1 cup baby spinach or kale
- 1 tablespoon chia seeds or ground flaxseeds
- 1 cup unsweetened coconut water or any non-dairy milk of your choice
- 1 tablespoon honey or pure maple syrup (optional)
- 1/2 teaspoon ground turmeric
- A pinch of ground black pepper
- A few ice cubes (optional)

Instructions:
1. In a blender, combine the chopped kiwifruit, cucumber, banana, baby spinach or kale, chia seeds or ground flaxseeds, coconut water or non-dairy milk, honey or maple syrup (if using), ground turmeric, and ground black pepper.
2. Blend on high speed until the mixture is smooth, creamy, and well combined. Add ice cubes if you prefer a colder and thicker texture.
3. Taste the smoothie and adjust the sweetness or seasoning as needed. If the smoothie is too thick, add a little more coconut water or non-dairy milk to achieve the desired consistency.
4. Pour the smoothie into two glasses and serve immediately. Enjoy this refreshing and nutritious smoothie for breakfast or as a snack.

Nutrients per serving:
- Calories: ~160 kcal
- Protein: ~4 g
- Fat: ~2 g
- Carbohydrates: ~36 g
- Fiber: ~6 g

Strawberry Beet Smoothie

Preparation time: 5 minutes
Servings: 2

Ingredients:
- 1 cup fresh or frozen strawberries
- 1 small beet, peeled and chopped
- 1 small banana, peeled and sliced
- 1 cup baby spinach or kale
- 1 tablespoon chia seeds or ground flaxseeds
- 1 cup unsweetened almond milk or any non-dairy milk of your choice
- 1 tablespoon honey or pure maple syrup (optional)
- 1/2 teaspoon ground turmeric
- A pinch of ground black pepper
- A few ice cubes (optional)

Instructions:
1. In a blender, combine the strawberries, chopped beet, banana, baby spinach or kale, chia seeds or ground flaxseeds, almond milk or non-dairy milk, honey or maple syrup (if using), ground turmeric, and ground black pepper.
2. Blend on high speed until the mixture is smooth, creamy, and well combined. Add ice cubes if you prefer a colder and thicker texture.
3. Taste the smoothie and adjust the sweetness or seasoning as needed. If the smoothie is too thick, add a little more almond milk or non-dairy milk to achieve the desired consistency.
4. Pour the smoothie into two glasses and serve immediately. Enjoy this refreshing and nutritious smoothie for breakfast or as a snack.

Nutrients per serving:
- Calories: ~180 kcal
- Protein: ~4 g
- Fat: ~4 g
- Carbohydrates: ~33 g
- Fiber: ~7 g

Green Goddess Detox Smoothie

Preparation time: 10 minutes
Servings: 1

Ingredients:
- 1 cup fresh spinach leaves
- 1/2 avocado, pitted and peeled
- 1/2 cucumber, chopped
- 1/2 cup fresh pineapple chunks
- 1/2 cup unsweetened almond milk
- 1/4 cup fresh parsley leaves
- 1/4 cup fresh mint leaves
- 1/2 lemon, juiced
- 1 tbsp chia seeds
- 1 tbsp fresh ginger, grated
- 1 cup ice

Instructions:
1. Place spinach, avocado, cucumber, pineapple, almond milk, parsley, mint, lemon juice, chia seeds, and grated ginger in a blender.
2. Blend on high until smooth and creamy.
3. Add the ice and blend again until the smoothie reaches your desired consistency.
4. Pour into a glass and enjoy immediately.

Nutrients per serving:
- Calories: ~230 kcal
- Protein: ~6 g
- Fat: ~11 g
- Carbohydrates: ~30 g
- Fiber: ~9 g

Pineapple Turmeric Twist Smoothie

Preparation time: 10 minutes
Servings: 1

Ingredients:
- 1 cup fresh or frozen pineapple chunks
- 1/2 banana
- 1/2 cup unsweetened coconut milk
- 1/2 cup Greek yogurt or dairy-free yogurt alternative
- 1 tsp freshly grated turmeric root or 1/4 tsp ground turmeric
- 1/2 tsp freshly grated ginger root or 1/4 tsp ground ginger
- 1/2 tsp ground cinnamon
- 1 tbsp chia seeds
- 1 tbsp honey or maple syrup (optional)
- 1 cup ice

Instructions:
1. Place pineapple, banana, coconut milk, yogurt, turmeric, ginger, cinnamon, chia seeds, and honey or maple syrup (if using) in a blender.
2. Blend on high until smooth and creamy.
3. Add the ice and blend again until the smoothie reaches your desired consistency.
4. Pour into a glass and enjoy immediately.

Nutrients per serving:
- Calories: ~270 kcal
- Protein: ~12 g
- Fat: ~10 g
- Carbohydrates: ~37 g
- Fiber: ~7 g

Frequently Asked Questions

In this chapter, you'll find answers to common questions that beginners often have when embarking on their Wall Pilates journey. Whether you're seeking clarification on certain aspects of the practice or wondering how to overcome challenges, this chapter aims to provide you with valuable insights and solutions to enhance your experience.

Q1: Can I practice Wall Pilates if I'm a beginner?

Absolutely! Wall Pilates is an ideal starting point for beginners. The wall provides support and stability, making it easier to learn and perform the exercises correctly.

Q2: Do I need special equipment for Wall Pilates?

Most Wall Pilates exercises require minimal or no equipment. All you need is a clear wall space and perhaps a yoga mat for added comfort.

Q3: How long should I hold each exercise?

The duration of each exercise can vary, but a good starting point is to hold each exercise for about 15-30 seconds. As you become more comfortable, you can gradually increase the duration.

Q4: Can I modify exercises if I find them too challenging?

Absolutely. Modification is key to accommodating your fitness level. If an exercise feels too challenging, consider using smaller movements or simplifying the movement pattern until you build strength and confidence.

Q5: How do I prevent straining my neck during exercises?

Focus on maintaining proper alignment and engaging your core. Keep your neck in line with your spine and avoid letting your head drop or hang. If you're unsure, consult the instructions for each exercise or seek guidance from a fitness professional.

Q6: How can I progress in Wall Pilates?

As you become more comfortable with the exercises, gradually increase the number of sets, repetitions, or duration. You can also explore more advanced variations of the exercises to continue challenging yourself.

Q7: Can Wall Pilates help with back pain?

Yes, Wall Pilates can be beneficial for back pain relief. The emphasis on core strength, posture, and flexibility can help alleviate back discomfort. However, if you have existing back issues, consult a healthcare provider before starting any new exercise program.

Q8: Is it normal to feel sore after Wall Pilates?

Yes, mild muscle soreness can be normal, especially if you're new to exercise or trying new movements. It's a sign that your muscles are adapting and getting stronger. Make sure to hydrate, rest, and continue with gentle movements to promote recovery.

Q9: How often should I progress to more advanced exercises?

There's no rush to progress. Listen to your body and gradually introduce more advanced exercises as you feel ready. It's essential to maintain proper form and avoid overexertion.

Q10: Can I practice Wall Pilates if I have specific medical conditions?

If you have any medical conditions or concerns, it's advisable to consult with your healthcare provider before starting a new exercise program, including Wall Pilates. They can provide personalized guidance based on your health situation.

Conclusion: Embrace Your Wall Pilates Journey

The journey into Wall Pilates is filled with curiosity, discovery, and growth. Your questions are a natural part of this process, and seeking answers is a testament to your commitment to your well-being. As you continue on this path, remember that every step, every question, and every practice session contributes to your overall progress. Feel free to revisit this chapter whenever you need guidance, and know that you're not alone on this journey. With dedication and patience, you'll uncover the transformative power of Wall Pilates in your life.

Conclusion

Your Journey with Wall Pilates

Congratulations on completing your exploration of Wall Pilates! You've embarked on a journey that has introduced you to the unique world of mindful movement, strength-building, and holistic well-being. Through the pages of this book, you've learned about the foundational principles of Wall Pilates, engaged in a variety of exercises, and discovered how to integrate this practice into your daily routine.

Your journey with Wall Pilates is not just about the physical movements; it's a journey of self-discovery, self-care, and personal growth. By practicing Wall Pilates, you've embraced the opportunity to connect with your body, cultivate mindfulness, and prioritize your health in a way that's sustainable and fulfilling.

As you move forward, keep these key takeaways in mind:

- **Start Where You Are:** Whether you're a beginner or have some fitness experience, Wall Pilates offers a supportive space to begin or continue your fitness journey.

- **Listen to Your Body:** Your body is your best guide. Pay attention to how you feel during exercises, and respect your limitations. Progress at your own pace.

- **Mindful Movement:** Embrace the art of mindful movement. Engage in each exercise with intention, focusing on your breath, alignment, and the sensations in your body.

- **Consistency Matters:** Consistency is the foundation of progress. Dedicate regular time to your Wall Pilates practice, and over time, you'll see and feel the results.

- **Versatility and Adaptability:** Wall Pilates can be tailored to your needs and preferences. Modify exercises, combine them with other forms of exercise, and make Wall Pilates a versatile part of your routine.

- **Holistic Wellness:** Your journey with Wall Pilates goes beyond physical fitness. It's an opportunity to nurture your mental and emotional well-being, creating a harmonious balance in your life.

Remember that your journey doesn't end here—it's an ongoing evolution. Continue to explore, learn, and refine your Wall Pilates practice as you grow stronger and more attuned to your body. Celebrate every achievement, no matter how small, and embrace the transformation that occurs both inside and out.

Thank you for choosing to embark on this journey with Wall Pilates. May the knowledge and experiences you've gained from this book guide you toward a life of vitality, mindfulness, and whole-body wellness. As you move forward, may your practice become a source of inspiration, empowerment, and joy! Your journey with Wall Pilates is a testament to your commitment to self-care and a healthier, happier you. Keep moving, keep breathing, and keep shining!

Printed in Great Britain
by Amazon

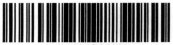

34635583R00066